NOTICES OF THE PRESS.

PHYSICIAN AND PATIENT; or, A PRACTICAL VIEW OF THE MUTUAL DUTIES, RELATIONS, AND INTERESTS OF THE MEDICAL PROFESSION AND THE COMMUNITY. By. W. Hooker, M.D.

We know of no other book that takes the intermediate space between the professional corps and the general reader, so as to be adapted to interest and profit equally both classes.—*Daily Chronicle, New London.*

It is a work of which the profession may not only be proud but thankful; and from which all may find hints for their own conduct.—*Literary World.*

We cannot forbear to add the expression of our pleasure at the successful manner in which the author has performed his task. His train of argument and illustrations are sound and logical, his facts apposite, and the purpose and style in which the whole is dressed, are in harmony with the subject, and well adapted to secure the continued attention of his readers. We hail the appearance of "Physician and Patient," as a valuable addition to our medical literature.—*Medical Examiner, Phila.*

We would strongly urge upon medical men to read the "Physician and Patient," and to pass it round the town or village, if perchance it may open the eyes of the great public to their own mental blindness.—*Boston Medical and Surgical Journal.*

No one can read this book without perceiving that its author is a sensible man and an experienced physician. It is not a professional work to be read merely by physicians—but a philosophical treatise on matters that are interesting to every one who has ever been ill, ever expects to be, or to have a friend suffering from disease in any of its forms.—*Boston Daily Advertiser.*

No physician can afford to do without it, nor have the public less interest in it.—*Newark Advertiser*

We have seldom met with a better specimen of sound, practical sense than that exhibited in this volume.—*The Presbyterian.*

The chief characteristic of the book is that it is replete with common sense.—*Norwich Courier.*

Dr. Hooker has, in his work, bestowed a just favor upon his profession and a great one upon the community.—*Springfield Gazette.*

We have no hesitation in commending this work as one of great value —*N Y. Observer.*

All must agree that it is written with undoubted ability, and that it contains a great deal of profitable instruction.—*Savannah Republican.*

The observations of an experienced practitioner, and eminently worthy of being read and attentively considered.—*Norwich Aurora.*

NOTICES OF THE PRESS.

Dr. Hooker has performed a good service to the public in presenting them with this book. He has exposed many of the impositions connected with modern quackery. Such a book was called for by the exigency of the times.—*Christian Intelligencer.*

It is full of wise instruction with regard to the reciprocal duties of physician and patient; of practical hints concerning the conduct and treatment of the sick, and judicious reflections on the ailments of both mind and body.—*Metropolis.*

We can hardly speak too highly of this work, and sincerely think that its circulation is adapted to correct many erroneous notions, and to minister to the health and comfort of the community.—*N. Y. Evangelist.*

A very excellent work, and one which should be in the hands of every member of the community. Dr. Hooker has done his work well.—*Hartford Republican.*

A capital exposure of empiricism in all its forms, and a faithful exhibition of the relative duties of physicians and patients.—*The Princeton Magazine.*

Such a mass of common sense, unmingled with anything irrelevant or captious, I have seldom, if ever, met with in so small a compass. There is not a solitary remark to which can even plausibly be applied the term, *telum imbelle sine ictu.* I wish the book could be placed in every family circle, and read, and pondered, and followed well and wisely, and thus prove, as I trust it will, a *Family Manual* in regard to the subjects on which it treats.—*Rev. George Upfold, D.D , Bishop of Indiana.*

This is a most readable and instructive volume.—*Home Journal.*

It bears the evidence of having been written with much care and reflection as well as ability.—*Portland Advertiser.*

It is written with decided ability.—*New-York Recorder.*

We like the design, and, as far as we have been able to examine it, the execution of this book very much.—*Central Christian Journal, Cincinnati.*

It is calculated to do good, and it will certainly give to its author a foremost place among the medical writers of the time.—*Boston Post.*

Those who desire the perusal of an entertaining book, containing most valuable instruction on a matter of the highest interest and importance, cannot do better than keep this volume on the parlor table, since it will not only bear frequent perusal, but will suggest matter of conversation after the usual inquiry of the health of the visitee.—*Evening Post, N. Y.*

It is written in a chaste, glowing, and vigorous style, and treats upon the subjects discussed with the usual common sense of the writer, and with a manliness, courtesy, and thoroughness, which must win for it not only the approval of the public, but an enviable reputation for the author.—*New-England Fountain.*

HOMŒOPATHY.

No. XIII.] [1851

Fiske Fund Prize Dissertation of the Rhode Island Medical Society.

HOMŒOPATHY:

AN EXAMINATION OF ITS DOCTRINES AND EVIDENCES.

BY

WORTHINGTON HOOKER, M. D.

AUTHOR OF "PHYSICIAN AND PATIENT," AND "MEDICAL DELUSIONS"

" Folly in wisdom hatch'd,
Hath wisdom's warrant, and the help of school."
LOVE'S LABOR LOST.

NEW YORK:

CHARLES SCRIBNER, 145 NASSAU STREET.

1851.

The Trustees of the Fiske Fund, at the Annual Meeting of the Rhode Island Medical Society, held at Providence, on the 25th of June, 1851, announced, that they had awarded to the author of the Dissertation bearing the motto,

"Folly in wisdom hatch'd,
Hath wisdom's warrant, and the help of school."

the premium of Fifty Dollars, by them offered for the best dissertation on the following subject, viz. :—

"HOMŒOPATHY, SO CALLED, ITS HISTORY AND REFUTATION."

Upon breaking the seal of the accompanying packet, they ascertained its author to be, WORTHINGTON HOOKER, M.D., of Norwich, Conn.

In awarding premiums, neither the Trustees, nor the Rhode Island Medical Society, hold themselves responsible for doctrines inculcated or opinions advanced.

GEORGE CAPRON,
HIRAM ALLEN,
WILLIAM A. SHAW. } Trustees.

(Attest,) S. AUGUSTUS ARNOLD, *Secretary*.

INTRODUCTION.

Absurd as Homœopathy appears on the face of it to the man of science or of plain common sense, the extent of its absurdity is revealed only by a thorough examination of its pretended facts and its plausible reasonings. Such an examination, it is obvious, is not given to it by the mass of those who believe in this vaunted system. A wordy and finespun theory, built upon the loosest analogies, especially if accompanied, as is usual with all forms of delusion and quackery, with reports of wonderful cures, is sufficient to satisfy them, at least till some other system presents itself, with similar appliances for fascinating the ear of popular credulity.

And it is not merely the novelty-seeking and the superficial who manifest this credulity; but we find many of the well-informed and intelligent, though they may be on their guard against errors and false theories on all other subjects, occasionally entrapped by delusions in medicine. For, although there is in the investigation of medicine a peculiar necessity for rigid observation and cautious reasoning, there is more disposition to observe carelessly and reason loosely on this subject, than there is in relation to any other in the wide range of science. This is to be seen even among those whose occupations favor the formation of good habits of observation and reasoning. The lawyer, who is in the habit of scrutinizing testimony, is apt to set aside his strict rules of evidence when he opens his ear to medical statements, and he forgets to sift them with the ingenious cross-questioning, with which he has so often elicited truth and unmasked falsehood in the court-room. The clergyman often gives credence to statements and dogmas in medicine, that are founded on proofs which he would scout as utterly fallacious if they were applied to theology, or indeed to any other subject. The scientific man, even though he may be engaged in some department of science, in which rigid demonstration and careful experimenting are constantly put in requisition, is often made a convert to some system of medicine, or even to some nostrum, by the force of loose analogies, or looser statements. The man of business too, who examines everything with his plain, shrewd common sense, and because he does so, succeeds where others less wary fail, dismisses this sentinel so faithful to warn of error, the moment that he enters the domain of medicine, and yields himself to the guidance of a blind credulity. Even the physician does not always go counter to the prevalent disposition of the community, but sometimes yields to the general tendency; and accordingly we have, in the records of medical experience a vast amount of careless and ill-digested observation and reasoning. The causes of this loose habit of mind in relation to medical subjects, it is not necessary here to trace out; but of its prevalence and of its wide influence in fostering delusion and quackery, the evidences are palpable and abundant.

The investigation, then, which I propose to make of Homœopathy in this essay, will be of service, not merely in putting a proper estimate upon the claims of this system to our belief; but also, and chiefly, in developing the true application of the rules of evidence to medical practice generally, and in exposing the various misapplications of them, which are the sources of so much error both in the popular and the professional mind. Medical delusions, generally, though so diversified in their forms, have a strong family resemblance, and the fallacies of Homœopathy may be considered as the types of other fallacies. An exposition of them, therefore, will reveal to the reader the foundations of other delusions and forms of quackery, and will perhaps enable him so to apply the principles of evidence in medicine, that he may in future the more readily detect error, whether it appear in the garb of learning or of ignorance.

A refutation merely of Homœopathy, without regard to other delusions, or to the general sources of error, would be a comparatively trivial, and almost useless effort. If it should be successful in dislodging this boasted system from its hold upon the popular belief and favor, some other fallacious system would take its place. And if left to itself, it would in a little time pass away, like all other delusions before it. In attacking Homœopathy therefore, we must look beyond this delusion, and aim at an exposure of the common sources of error, if we wish to produce any valuable and permanent effect.

The examination of Homœopathy presented in this essay, will, I trust, commend itself to my readers as being fair and candid. I have no desire to search out its weak points, and leave untouched its strong ones, if there be any; but I am willing to meet it at every point. I have endeavored to look at the subject as a whole, and not take any partial view of it. I have also endeavored to discover the exact positions of the various writers on Homœopathy, so that I may not misstate the views of any one. I have been the more careful on this point, because Homœopathists are so prone to make abundant use of any accidental misrepresentation of their doctrines, however slight it may be; and thus divert attention from the real and main points at issue. Whatever is at all doubtful I have omitted, and have taken into view only those points on which the statements and reasonings of Homœopathic writers are most explicit and clear. I have found many discrepancies and inconsistencies between different prominent Homœopathists, some of which I notice. It will be seen that I do not make Homœopathy responsible for everything which has been said for it by its advocates; but that I am willing even to strip it of all in regard to which there is any disagreement among them, and let its merits stand or fall by an examination of what remains.

Homœopathy is so absurd, that it seems almost a waste of time and effort to go through with a formal refutation of it. And so it would be, were its refutation not made necessary, from its adoption by so many of the intelligent and influential among the non-medical portion of the community. Such persons, I trust, will find, on reading this essay, that their belief in the system of Hahnemann has been formed without a real understanding of its merits. And I flatter myself that those of them who will give me a candid hearing, will be induced to abandon such a combination of falsities and inconsistencies as this system presents.

Homœopathists complain that physicians ridicule their doctrines, and very gravely say, that the system of the "sage of Coethen," is not to be put down by a laugh. But when things are exceedingly laughable, it is a little unreasonable to demand of us an imperturbable gravity. When Homœopathy conjures up its ridiculous fantasies to play before us like so many harlequins, it is hard to be denied the privilege of laughing at them. As to the alleged impropriety of ridicule in the discussion of the merits of this system, it may be remarked, that it cannot be improper if it only be used fairly; and if a little pleasantry suffice to demolish an error, it surely is an unnecessary waste of power to attack it with strong and sober argument. It were folly to deal sturdy blows at bubbles which can be dissolved by the slightest touch.

With these few preliminary remarks, I invite the reader to accompany me in this examination; and if he will take the pains to go to the sources from which I have derived my information in regard to the doctrines of Homœopathy, I shall be glad to have my accuracy put to this test. The authorities upon which I have relied are solely standard Homœopathic authors. I have selected the best of them, so far as I could find by enquiring of Homœopathists themselves which are the best. I have not undertaken to go through all the Homœopathic literature that could be found, for that would be a waste of time, to say nothing of the toilsomeness and disgust attending such a pilgrimage. A list of the authorities to which I refer, may be found at the conclusion of this essay.

W. HOOKER.

NORWICH, CONN., *August*, 1851.

CONTENTS.

CHAPTER I.

EXPOSITION OF THE SYSTEM OF HAHNEMANN.

CHAPTER II.

EXPOSITION OF THE SYSTEM OF HAHNEMANN, CONTINUED.

CHAPTER III.

EXAMINATION OF THE DOCTRINES OF HOMŒOPATHY.

CHAPTER IV.

EXAMINATION OF THE DOCTRINES OF HOMŒOPATHY, CONTINUED.

CHAPTER V.

PRACTICAL EVIDENCES OF HOMŒOPATHY.

CHAPTER VI.

ESTIMATE OF HAHNEMANN

CHAPTER VII.

CONCLUDING OBSERVATIONS.

HOMŒOPATHY.

CHAPTER I.

EXPOSITION OF THE SYSTEM OF HAHNEMANN.

Samuel Hahnemann, the founder of the system termed Homœopathy, was born at Messein, in Saxony, in the year 1755. His father was a painter on porcelain, and had not the means of giving him a professional education. "Happily, however," says Mr. Sampson, one of his warmest eulogists, "at twelve years of age he attracted the attention of Dr. Muller, the Director of the Provincial School, by whom a free admission was procured for him to all the advantages of that establishment. His progress was rapid, and in a short time he became one of the assistant teachers." On leaving this school, he resolved to devote himself to the medical profession. For this purpose he went to the university of Leipsic, with only twenty ducats in his pocket. He supported himself there by translating French and English works into German. At the end of two years he went to Vienna, to gain in the hospitals of that city the advantages of extensive practical observation. He there, Mr. Sampson informs us, obtained the favor of Dr Quarin, Physician to the Emperor of Austria; and the Governor of Hermandstadt having afterward made him the medical attendant of his household, he, in that post, acquired a sufficient sum to enable him to return to Germany, where, in 1779, he took the degree of M.D. at the university of Erlangen.

Hahnemann now settled as a practitioner of medicine in Dresden, and in 1785 he married Henriette Kuchler, the daughter of a chemist. He was quite a large contributor to the medical periodicals at this time; and he published some works, which his eulogists pronounced to be very remarkable. Though his prospects of success were very flattering, it is said that he was so much dissatisfied with the uncertainty attending the practice of medicine then in vogue, that he relinquished his profession, and devoted himself to the study of chemistry, and to the translation of foreign works.

"At length," says Mr. Sampson, "in the year 1790, whilst translating the Materia Medica of Cullen, being struck with the contradictory statements which it contained regarding the action of Peruvian bark upon the human system, it occurred to him to test the action of this medicine upon himself. The first dose produced symptoms similar to those of the peculiar kind of intermittent fever which the same medicine is known to cure; and his attention having been strongly arrested by this fact, he repeated the experiment, and also induced some friends to resort to a similar trial, in order to ascertain that it was not accidental. The results in each case were confirmatory of the first; and the question seems to have been irresistibly forced upon him, "Can it be possible that this property which I now observe in Peruvian bark, of producing symptoms analogous to those of the disease for which it is a remedy, is a property peculiar to medicines of all kinds? From that moment he commenced a series of experiments on other substances—mercury, belladonna, digitalis, cocculus, etc., which, in proportion as he extended them, led him to the conviction that his supposition had really embraced a universal therapeutic law."

It was not, however, till 1796, six years after this, that he published his first dissertation on Homœopathy in Hufeland's Journal; and it was not till 1805, that he issued his first formal work on the subject. The next year he published another work entitled, "Medicine Founded on Experience," forming the basis of his famous "Organon of the Healing Art," which was put forth complete in the year 1810. So confident had he now become of the truth of his doctrine, that he boldly declares in his preface, "The true art of healing remained undiscovered until my time." In 1811 he began the publication of a very extensive work, his "Materia Medica Pura," which was not completed till ten years had elapsed.

Having removed to Leipsic, he, in 1812, delivered a course of lectures, and began to gather around him believers in his doctrine. But, it is said by his eulogists, that the physicians and apothecaries of Leipsic were very soon arrayed against him in active hostility, and that, at length, with the aid of the profession in Dresden, they obtained an order from government for the enforcement of an obsolete law, which prohibits physicians from preparing or dispensing their own medicines. So much did the success of Homœopathy depend in Hahnemann's view upon the careful preparation of the medicines, that he now "saw himself compelled to relinquish practice, or to endanger the real progress of his system, by entering into a compromise with his opponents." He adopted the former alternative, and publicly announced his intention to relinquish practice. The persecution to which he was subjected, made his doctrines spread rapidly; and the Duke of Anhalt Coethen, having become one of his admirers, offered him an asylum from his persecutors. He removed, therefore, to Coethen, and in 1821 was made one of the duke's councillors.

This part of Hahnemann's history may, for aught that I know, be true; but the story is certainly a very singular one. It is strange that no one of his adherents could be found willing and competent to act as his apothecary. And stranger still is it that, after having come so deliberately to the firm belief that he had discovered the true art of healing, he should at the first show of opposition be frightened into a relinquishment of the practice of the art. A higher courage, and a more indomitable perseverance than this indicates, are surely to be looked for in one who is conscious of having discovered in medicine "the great gift of God to man."

While Hahnemann resided at Coethen, he published, in 1812, a work on chronic diseases, in four volumes. In 1827 his wife died. After remaining a widower nearly eight years, he married Mademoiselle Melanie d'Hervilly, a French lady who visited Coethen in order to consult him. Though he was now eighty years old, he bade farewell to Coethen, and removed with his new bride to busy Paris. Here he practiced Homœopathy until his death, which occurred in 1843, in the eighty-ninth year of his age.

There is one fact in the history of Hahnemann, which is never alluded to by his admirers. In the early part of his career he appeared before the public as the seller of secret nostrums. "About the year 1800," says Dr. Leo Wolf, "Hahnemann advertised a new salt, of which he claimed the discovery, and which he sold at the modest price of a *louis d'or* per ounce. The Society for the Promotion of Natural Sciences, desirous of becoming acquainted with this new substance, had it analyzed by some of the most experienced chemists, who pronounced it to be nothing but common borax. He shortly afterward advertised an infallible preventive of scarlet fever; but being disappointed in its sale, he afterward confessed it to be nothing but a few grains of extract of belladonna dissolved in water." These transactions brand "the sage of Coethen" not only as a mercenary quack, but as a dishonest one.

If the great central doctrine of Hahnemann's system, *similia similibus curantur*, be true, the "sage of Coethen" is fully entitled to a place in the ranks of discoverers in medicine. True, this doctrine had been hinted at before, time and again ; and the fanciful Stahl, who flourished in the last of the seventeenth century, announced it in the following explicit language : "The received method in medicine of treating diseases by opposite remedies, that is to say, by medicines which are opposed to the effects they produce, is completely false and absurd. I am persuaded, on the contrary, that diseases are subdued by agents which produce a similar affection—burns by the heat of a fire to which the parts are exposed ; the frost-bite by snow or icy cold water ; and inflammations and contusions by spirituous applications." This sounds very much like the language of Hahnemann himself. But still, up to the time of Hahnemann, no one, not even Stahl, thought of promulgating the doctrine, *similia similibus curantur* as the basis of a system of medicine—as the "sole law of cure" in all diseases. If what Hahnemann teaches in regard to it be true, then clearly it is not merely the development of the bare truth, but the revealing of the mode and the scope of its application, and the collecting of all the proofs which bear upon it, that entitle him to the honored appellation of discoverer. Dairymen and dairywomen, in great numbers, saw that the vaccine disease was a preventive of smallpox long before Jenner knew it. But this does not at all detract from his merit as a discoverer; for Jenner was the first to see the wide scope of the fact, to collect the proofs of it, and to indicate the exact way in which it should be used as a preventive.

But whatever may be said of Hahnemann's right of discovery in regard to the great central doctrine of his system, there were other doctrines taught by him, in relation to which this right is beyond a question—they were wholly original with him. The doctrine that infinitesimal doses of medicine are adequate to the cure of disease—a doctrine, which, if true, is one of the most valuable and wonderful of all discoveries—was never suggested even in the most dim and remote manner to any mind. The honor of this discovery, if it be one, belongs exclusively to the "Sage of Coethen." And then, too, the doctrine that psora (vulgarly called the itch) is the cause of seven eighths of all the cases of chronic disease in the world, was, certainly, not among the things "dreamt of" in any one's philosophy till Hahnemann arose.

I now invite the attention of the reader to an exposition of the system of Hahnemann, as developed in his "Organon"—a work which is universally regarded by Homœopathists as the great text-book of medicine.

I give from this work what he terms "a short analysis of the Homœopathic method." After going through with one hundred and sixty pages of fanciful, though rather ingenious reasoning, founded upon both loose and false statements and mere analogies, he thus sums up:

"From all that has been here stated, the following truths must be admitted:

"1st. There is nothing for the physician to cure in disease but the sufferings of the patient, and the changes in his state of health, which are perceptible to the senses, that is to say, the totality or mass of symptoms by which the disease points out the remedy it stands in need of—every internal cause that could be attributed to it—every occult character that man might be tempted to bestow, are nothing more than so many idle dreams and vain imaginings.

"2d. That state of the organism which we call disease, cannot be converted into health but by the aid of another affection of the organism excited by means of medicines.* The experiments made upon healthy individuals are the best and purest means that could be adopted to discover this virtue.

"3d. According to every known fact, it is impossible to cure a natural disease by the aid of medicines which have the faculty of producing a contrary artificial state or symptom in healthy persons. There-

* This is very explicit: no cure is effected by anything but medicine. *Nature* is out of the question. And yet Hahnemann does allow in other places, and even upon the very next page, that nature sometimes cures a disease by substituting another similar one in its place. But this, he thinks, is seldom done; for it is effected, he says (p. 141), only through the agency of "miasmatic diseases, such as psora, measles, and small-pox." And he remarks that "nature can cure but a very limited number of diseases with these hazardous remedies."

fore, the Allopathic method can never effect a real cure. Even nature never performs a cure, or annihilates one disease by adding to it another that is dissimilar, be the intensity of the latter ever so great.

"4th. Every fact serves to prove that a medicine capable of exciting in healthy persons a morbid symptom dissimilar to the disease that is to be cured, never effects any other than momentary relief in disease of long standing without curing it, and suffers it to re-appear after a certain interval, more aggravated than ever. The Antipathic and purely palliative method is, therefore, wholly opposed to the object that is to be attained where the disease is an important one and of long standing.

5th. The third method, the only one to which we can still have recourse (the Homœopathic), which employs against the totality of the symptoms of a natural disease, a medicine that is capable of exciting in healthy persons symptoms that closely resemble those of the disease itself, is the only one that is really salutary, and which always annihilates disease, or the purely dynamic aberrations of the vital powers in an easy, prompt, and perfect manner. In this respect nature herself furnishes the example when, by adding to an existing disease a new one that resembles it, she cures it promptly and effectually."

The reader sees that Hahnemann recognizes three modes of treating disease—the Antipathic, Allopathic, and Homœopathic. The Antipathic (taking its name from ἀντι opposite, and, πάθος suffering or disease) consists in producing effects opposite in character to the symptoms of the disease to be overcome. The use of opium in producing sleep in the restless and wakeful, and in giving ease to the suffering, is an example of this method. Hahnemann boldly asserts, in face of the experience of ages, that this method only palliates for the moment, and *never* cures. The Allopathic* method (deriving its name from ἄλλος, another, and πάθος) consists in producing effects altogether different from, though not opposite to, the symptoms of disease. Of this method Hahnemann says that "without ever regarding that which is really diseased in the body, it attacks those parts which are sound, in order to draw off the malady from another quarter, and direct it toward the latter." He says, also, that this method "cannot cure in any

* The term Allopathist, which the followers of Hahnemann apply to every physician of the regular profession, it must be obvious to the reader, is entirely inappropriate. Physicians employ the Antipathic as well as the Allopathic mode of treating disease, and it would be as proper to style them Antipathists as Allopathists. Besides, physicians employ many remedies which relieve disease after a mode which is as yet not at all understood. However, for the sake of *convenience*, I shall use the terms Allopathic and Allopathist in the senses which Homœopathists ordinarily attach to them.

I see that some of the later Homœopathic writers, as Dr. Joslin, for example, say Allœopathic instead of Allopathic. In this case the derivation is from ἀλλοῖος (not ἄλλος), to correspond with the ὁμοῖος of Homœopathy. As the term is altogether a misnomer, and as I consent to its use merely for convenience' sake, I shall leave the question of derivations to our Homœopathic friends who are so fond of formidable words of classical origin, and shall adopt the term as most commonly used, and not burden a word already sufficiently long with another syllable.

case; having no analogy, or opposing force to the symptoms of the disease, it can never reach the parts affected; it may suspend the symptoms for a time by heterogeneous suffering, but it cannot destroy them." You have a familiar example of this method in the application of a blister to relieve internal inflammation or irritation. In this case the disease is removed by producing another disease upon one of "those parts which are sound"—the skin. The Homœopathic method (so termed from ὁμοῖος, like, and πάθος) consists in producing effects analogous to, or very nearly resembling the symptoms of the disease. This method Hahnemann says "is the only one which experience proves to be always salutary. The pure and specific effects of the remedies employed being perfectly analogous to the natural symptoms, *they go right to the parts affected;* and as two similar diseases cannot exist at the same time in the same system, the natural symptoms give way, provided the artificial ones slightly surpass them in intensity."

In this summary of Hahnemann's conclusions or "analysis of the Homœopathic method (as he calls it) the reader will notice that there is nothing said about infinitesimal doses. And it is remarkable that there is not the slightest hint upon this subject in the Organon till we reach the 204th page, though the whole book contains but 300 pages, and then it is alluded to only in a note, and that merely incidentally. Almost all that he does say about it from beginning to end is said in notes. In the text it is not treated of at all in any explicit and circumstantial manner, but is barely hinted at. Yet Hahnemann and his followers uniformly speak of his alleged discovery of the efficacy of infinitesimals as a very great achievement in medical science. And most surely, if it be a real discovery, it is one which should excite our wonder and admiration as a most singular and stupendous discovery.

The ideas which prevail among even the believers of Homœopathy in regard to the minuteness of infinitesimal doses are very indefinite; and when physicians make statements in relation to them, most persons think that they are indulging in a little playful extravagance at the expense of a very worthy class of men, and that Homœopathic physicians do not really give such extremely small doses as Allopathists say that they do. I shall therefore endeavor to give the reader as definite an idea as it is possible to do of the extent to which Homœopathists carry their attenuations. This will be somewhat difficult. The Arithmetic of Homœopathy goes beyond all chemistry—no test can reach its higher dilutions. And not only so, but its calculations have to do with figures which defy even our conceptions. On this point Dr Forbes well says, "The *hundredth* part of a grain is intelligible enough; the *ten thousandth* is comprehensible, but begins to waver before the mental view; while the millionth part of a grain puts our powers of comprehension on the rack, and leaves us in a chaos of undefined entities, or nonentities, we know not which. We fancy that we grasp the reality, and then it instantly vanishes as a phantom, even beyond the sphere of imagination itself. Having got so far, the additional subdivisions or attenuations scarcely add to our difficulties. The mind in any such case is occupied by a word more than a thing, and whether the word be a millionth, billionth, or decillionth, the power of comprehension seems the same. And yet the *actual difference* between these quantities is immense,—so immense as to be almost as inconceivable as the actual things themselves."

In the calculations which I shall attempt to make in this towering arithmetic, I shall try to be accurate. But if I should accidentally commit any error involving such trifling amounts as millions or billions, I trust the reader will pardon me, for I shall only be following the example of Homœopathists, who, as you will see in another part of this essay, make nothing of jumping millions, billions, trillions, etc., etc., in dosing their patients.

If I should tell one who, though a believer in Homœopathy, has never been initiated into the mysteries of Hahnemannic arithmetic, that a grain of any article highly attenuated would be sufficient to supply all the Homœopathic physicians in the world with all which they would want to use of that article in a whole year, he would consider it a wild, over statement. If I should tell him that this falls very far short of the truth, and that if Homœopathy had been the universal practice from Adam till now, not a grain of any one medicine, if administered in any of the higher attenuations, could have been used up by this time, he would consider it a most extravagant libel upon Homœopathy. And then if I should go farther, and tell him, that if medicine be given in the thirtieth dilution (in doses from which Homœopathists profess to witness appreciable results, even in the case of such substances as charcoal and oystershell); and, if all the inhabitants of the earth should take from one single grain thus attenuated, three or four doses daily, generation after generation, and if the population of the earth should remain the same that it is now, the grain would not be all gone till the lapse of about a sextillion of years, a period extending probably far, very far, beyond the millenium, or even the end of the world—such a statement would, if he gave it a thought, prompt him to say to me—'Ridiculous! You must be joking. It cannot be that my physician gives medicine in this way—he is too sensible a man for that. A grain of oystershell as medicine last the world through all time! Does Hahnemann really teach this, and do such men as Professor Henderson and Professor Joslin believe it?' And if I should assure him over and over again, that the climax which I had reached was just the truth in regard to the general practice of Homœopathists, and that some even go farther than this, he would still be disposed to think that I was imposing rather largely upon his credulity, and would very probably call for the proof of my assertions.

The truth is, that the employers of Homœopathic

physicians have never really looked into the arithmetic of the science, and do not know how much they are called upon to believe. Much is said of small doses, but no definite idea is given of the degree of their smallness; and, as will be seen in another part of this essay, the comparisons which are made by Homœopathic writers are calculated to blind and mislead on this very point.

The reader will obtain some idea of the minuteness of the Homœopathic attenuations by observing the processes by which they are made.

Hahnemann's description of his mode of preparing vegetable medicines (which I find in his Materia Medica Pura, vol. i. p. 96,) is as follows:—"To obtain the hundredth degree of potency, mix two drops of alcohol with equal parts of the juice of the plant, and then mix this with ninety-nine or one hundred drops of alcohol, by means of two strokes with the arm from above *downwards;* by mixing in the same way one drop of this dilution with one hundred drops of alcohol, you obtain the ten thousandth degree of potency, and by mixing a drop of this last dilution with another one hundred drops of alcohol you obtain the millionth degree. This process of spiritualization or dynamization is continued through a series of thirty phials up to the thirtieth solution. This thirtieth degree should always be used for Homœopathic purposes."

It will be seen that at each change from one phial to another, ninety-nine parts out of the hundred are thrown away. When the thirtieth phial is reached, each drop in that phial contains only a decillionth of a drop of the medicine which was in the first phial ; and this quantity is expressed by 1 for a numerator, and 1 with a string of sixty cyphers for a denominator.

Let us try to get some idea of the minuteness of this dilution. Let us see what quantities of liquid would be required for the successive dilutions, if instead of throwing away ninety-nine parts out of every hundred, the whole is retained. For the first dilution one hundred drops of alcohol would be used. For the second it would take ten thousand drops, or about a pint. For the third it would take one hundred pints. For the fourth ten thousand pints. And now it mounts up rapidly at each dilution. For the ninth dilution it would take ten billion of gallons, which, according to the computation of Dr. Panvani, equals the quantity of water in the Lake Agnano, which is two miles in circumference. For the twelfth dilution a million of such lakes would be required, or as it is reckoned by Dr. Post of New York, (from whom I shall take the liberty to borrow the remaining calculations rather than attempt them myself) it would require five hundred lakes as large as Lake Superior. The fifteenth dilution would require a quantity of alcohol greater in bulk than the earth. The eighteenth would require a quantity greater than the volume of the sun. And the thirtieth, the one which Hahnemann insists upon as being the best for common use, would take a quantity of alcohol exceeding the volume of a quadrillion of suns.*

But I find that adventurous as this arithmetic is, we have not yet reached the outmost boundary of these wonders. After the thirtieth dilution is made, the medicine is not even then ready for use. It must go through with another dilution still. Hahnemann tells us in a little note at the bottom of the page, that he exhibits "one globule of the size of a grain of flaxseed, three hundred of which weigh a grain.†

* The following jeu d'esprit, which appeared in a newspaper, so far from being a caricature, as the reader will see, falls very far short of the absurdity of Homœopathy. It is a prescription for a Homœopathic rum cordial.

Take a little rum,
The less you take the better;
Pour it in the lakes
Of Wener and of Wetter.

Dip a spoonful out,
Mind you don't get groggy,
Pour it in the lake
Winnipissiogee.

Stir the mixture well,
Lest it prove inferior,
Then put half a drop
Into Lake Superior.

Every other day
Take a drop in water,
You'll be better soon,
Or at least you ought to.

Attenuated as the dilution here described is, it falls very far short of the higher attenuations of Homœopathy, and especially that which is in so common use, the thirtieth dilution.

† I believe that the globules as ordinarily given, are of such a size that

One drop being sufficient to moisten upwards of a thousand such globules, one globule contains less than the one thousandth part of a drop of the decilionth solution." And to crown all, he tells us in another note, which the reader will find on the 298th page of the Organon, that "if the patient is very sensitive, it will be sufficient to let him smell once to a phial which contains a globule." And then he remarks, "after the patient has smelled to it, the phial is to be recorked, which will thus serve for years without its medicinal virtues being perceptibly impaired."*

But some, if possible, go even beyond this. I find it stated in Hull's Laurie, that "Hahnemann, in his latter years, was much in favor of an extension of the scale of potencies; and Gross and other continental homœopathists of repute have recently spoken strongly

it takes only twenty-five to weigh a grain, so that a common Homœopathic globule contains twelve times as much medicine as the true Hahnemannic globule, if it contain any, which is a good deal of a question. This, however, is a very trifling discrepancy for these Homœopathists; for, as you will see in another part of this essay, when they get up among the higher attenuations, it seems to be all the same whether they give the patient a globule moistened with the three hundreth part of a decillionth of a drop, or a dose containing millions upon millions of this quantity of the medicine.

* Hahnemann speaks of a preparation of gold so attenuated, that each grain contains only the quadrillionth part of a grain of the gold, in which by means of the rubbings, the medicinal virtue of the gold is "so developed, that it will be sufficient to put one grain of it into a phial, and to cause a melancholy person whose disgust of life has brought him to the verge of suicide, to breathe it for a few seconds, when *in one hour* (not more nor less I suppose) the wretched being will be relieved from the wicked demon, and restored to a relish of life."

of the striking results obtained from Arsenicum and other medicines at the two hundreth and even the eighteen hundredth attenuation!" This last attenuation is so very dilute, that it would require in its preparation, if none were thrown away, a quantity of alcohol exceeding the volume of the visible universe. Laurie remarks upon this that "their opinions and recommendations, *being derived from experience*, are at all events well worthy of considerate attention and careful investigation, whatever the *material-headed reasoners* may say to the contrary."

But enough of these airy flights, at least for the present. Most of my readers, I suppose, are "*material-headed* reasoners," and have never had their brains refined, etherealized in the laboratory of Hahnemann, and they must be getting dizzy by this time mid the whirl of "spiritualized" and "dynamized" atoms. I shall dismiss then for the present all farther calculations in the arithmetic of Homœopathy, and shall recur to the subject again when I come to speak of the range of doses employed by different Homœopathists.

How is it, the reader will ask, that these excessively minute doses act—by what virtue do they produce an effect upon the system? Hahnemann says that a new power is given to medicine by agitation and trituration. "Medicines," he asserts, (p. 295) "acquire at each division or dilution a new degree of power by the rubbing or shaking they undergo, a means of developing the inherent virtues of medicines that was unknown till my time; and which is so energetic, that latterly I have been forced by experience to reduce the number of shakes to two, of which I formerly prescribed ten to each dilution." He is extremely careful on this point. He cautions again and again against giving too many shakes,* and prescribes the exact manner in which the shakes should be made. It must be done with "a powerful stroke of the arm *descending*." (p. 300.) So in the preparation of powders he says that care must be taken "not to rub them down too much in the mortar." Thus in mixing one grain of any remedy with one hundred grains of sugar of milk, he says, (p. 300) "it ought to be rubbed down with force during one hour only, and the same space of time should not be exceeded in the subsequent dilutions, in order that the power of medicine may not be carried to too great an extent." The power communicated by this potentization, as it is termed, he speaks of as a "*spiritual* virtue," and

* "One drop of drosera," says Hahnemann, "diluted thirty times, each of which dilutions has been shaken twenty times, put in jeopardy the life of an infant to whom it was given; while the same medicine, when each dilution has received only *two* shakes, given in a quantity just sufficient to moisten a globule of sugar of the size of a grain of millet, will cure the disease easily and promptly." If twenty shakes at each dilution, that is six hundred in the whole, impart such *dangerous* potency to medicine, why is it that "Jenichen's High Potencies," which are recommended as having received a *million and a half* of shakes, so powerful as to produce a "metallic ringing sound of the glass bottle," are such mild and innocent remedies? One would suppose that they would not merely "put in jeopardy" the lives of the sick, but would kill outright.

similar language is very common among almost all Homœopathists. Even an article, which in its common form has from its insolubility no medicinal virtue, silex, for example, can be "potentized," he claims, by trituration and shaking, and thus be endued with such power, that a single grain of it would suffice, if thus prepared, to cure of certain forms of disease not merely a world of human beings, but millions upon millions of worlds peopled as thickly as our own.

CHAPTER II.

EXPOSITION OF THE SYSTEM OF HAHNEMANN, CONTINUED.

I WILL now give the reader as clear an idea as I can of the manner in which Hahnemann supposes that the minute doses cure disease. He asserts that medicines in the ordinary doses used by physicians "are not applied to the suffering parts themselves, but merely to those not attacked by the disease." Homœopathic medicines, on the contrary, he says, go directly to the parts which are diseased. I will quote his own language. "However feeble," he says, (p. 296) "the dose of a remedy may be, provided it can in the slightest degree aggravate the state of the patient homœopathically, provided it has the power of exciting symptoms similar to those of the primitive disease but rather more intense, it will in preference, and almost exclusively, affect those parts of the organism that are already in a state of suffering, and which are strongly irritated and predisposed to receive any irritation analogous to their own. Thus an artificial disease rather more intense is substituted in place of the natural one. The organism no longer suffers but from the former affection, which by reason of its nature and the minuteness of the dose by which it was produced, soon yields to the efforts of the vital force to restore the normal state, and thus leaves the body (if the disease was an acute one) free from suffering—that is to say in a healthy condition."

Let me paraphrase a little—and I wish the reader to compare the paraphrase critically with the original.

The process of cure as above described is this. The little dose, if chosen aright—that is, if the medicine is capable of producing in a healthy person symptoms similar to those of the disease to be attacked—has from this fact a peculiar affinity for the diseased part, and goes directly to it, and introduces into it a disease similar to the one to be dislodged. The "artificial disease" succeeds in dislodging the disease which it finds there, because it is a little stronger, or as Hahnemann has it, a "little more intensè." What now becomes of the new lodger thus introduced by the infinitesimal? Does it remain there as a permanent resident? No—it exercises but a *brief* authority. Its occupation is soon gone. "The vital force," that good guardian angel that old Cullen called the *vis medicatrix naturæ* at once turns out the usurper for two very good reasons—because it is so much like the previous occupant, and because it was introduced by such a little fellow.

Hahnemann scouts the idea of employing several remedies at once to dislodge a disease. Only one must be used at a time. One strong man armed if fitted for the purpose, though it be an exceedingly little one, can drive out the most powerful of diseases, however formidably it may be fortified in its position. No matter how violent the malady—the patient may have a burning fever, tumultuously may the blood run through its channels, excruciating may be the pain, raving the delirium, unceasing and extreme the restlessness—the magic infinitesimal finds its way to the very seat of the disease, and in the most quiet manner dispossesses it, putting in its place another disease, which though "more powerful" than the one it displaces, is yet so gentle, that the "vital force" makes an easy conquest, and establishes again the serene and happy dominon of health. What delightful Therapeutics!

Hahnemann and his followers seem to regard diseases as the merest playthings in their hands, doing as if by a charm, the bidding of their potentized infinitosimals. "When," says Hahnemann, "a proper application of the Homœopathic remedy has been made, the disease which is to be cured, however malignant and painful it may be, subsides in a *few hours*, if recent, and in a *few days* if it is already of long standing. Every trace of indisposition vanishes, and health is restored by a speedy and almost insensible transition." Even the eruptive diseases need not to run their course, but can be at once arrested and cured by the magic of Homœopathy. Hering in his Domestic Physician says of so severe and loathsome a malady as small pox, that it "is so easily cured by one or a couple of doses of Sulph. or Rhus, that this disease should no longer excite any uneasiness."

I will now call your attention to the manner in which Homœopathists discover to what disease any remedy has that peculiar affinity which is an essential condition of its curative power. It is done in this way. The remedy is given to persons in health. The symptoms which follow in them are carefully and minutely noted down. After making out this group of symptoms, you may be sure, as they say, that in whatever case you find a similar group of symptoms, there you have the disease which this remedy in infinitesimal doses will cure.

But by what rules, you will ask, are Homœopathists guided in ascertaining the symptoms? There is no formal set of rules prescribed, although the science of their Therapeutics is claimed to be an exceedingly refined and accurate science; and we are left to *infer* for the most part what the principles are which govern observers in conducting these "provings," as they are termed. The mode in which they are conducted, however, I will develope to the reader as clearly and faithfully as I can from the loose and scattered hints which I find in Homœopathic books on this subject.

I find nothing very definite in regard to the *size* of the doses used in these provings. Hahnemann's provings of Cinchona were made, at first, at least, with the ordinary doses of the common practice, and in his Organon he continually refers to the effects of such doses to prove his doctrines. But Dr Forbes says that the doses which he administered, at least in the later and principal trials, were infinitesimals. And this is probably true. For though he says in the text (p. 203) that "the dose is the same as that which practitioners are in the habit of prescribing in their ordinary recipes," he informs us in a note at the bottom of the page, "recently I have judged it more proper to administer only doses that are very weak and extenuated to a very high degree." The truth of the whole matter is, that it makes so little difference to Hahnemann and his followers whether the doses in the provings be infinitesimal or are in the "coarse form" used by "*ordinary* physicians," that they do not in their records of these provings indicate in any way the kind of doses with which they were made. Nothing definite is said in regard to this point in any of the books which I have consulted.

The person on whom a proving of any medicine is made must submit to certain restrictions of diet and regimen. I quote Hahnemann's language. "During the whole time of this experiment the diet must be extremely moderate. It is necessary to abstain as much as possible from spices, and to make use of nothing but simple food that is merely nourishing, carefully avoiding all green vegetables, roots, sallads, and soups with herbs, all of which, notwithstanding the preparations they have undergone, are aliments that still retain some small medicinal energy that disturbs the effect of the medicine. The drink is to remain the same as that in daily use, taking care that it is as little stimulating as possible."

"The person on whom this experiment is tried, ought to avoid all fatiguing labor of mind and body, all excesses, debauches, or mental excitement during the whole of the time that it continues" (p. 202).

The object of these restrictions is to withdraw everything from the subject of the trial "which will exercise a medicinal influence" upon him. The same restrictions are to be observed in administering to the sick; and as Hahnemann specifies the things to be avoided, more particularly under this head, I will transcribe the list for my readers.

"Coffee, tea, beer, containing vegetable substances that are not fit for the patient; liquors prepared from medicinal aromatics, chocolate, spices, sweet waters, and perfumery of all kinds; preparations for the teeth, either in powder or liquid, where medicinal substances are included; perfumed bags, strongly seasoned viands, pastry, and ice with spices; vegetables consisting of medicinal herbs and roots, old cheese, stale meat, pork, goose, duck, and young veal.* Every one of

* It is a little singular that so medicinal an article as tobacco is not in the excluded list. Perhaps the impossibility of excluding it in practice is the reason. It would be rather dangerous to the popularity of the new practice to interfere with a habit so prevalent as the use of tobacco. As I write this note a friend says that he believes that this is really one of the excluded articles. If so, it is rather strange that the great exemplar, while he was so particular as to mention such things as old cheese, pork, goose, sweet waters, perfumed bags, etc., should forget to mention an article so much more medicinal as tobacco is.

these act medicinally, and ought to be carefully removed from the patient. All abuses or excesses at table are to be interdicted, even the use of sugar, salt, and spirituous liquors; the physician will, likewise, forbid too warm apartments, sedentary life, passive exercise in riding or driving, sleeping after dinner, nocturnal amusements, uncleanliness, unnatural voluptuousness, and the reading of obscene books; we are likewise to avoid the causes of anger, grief, and malice, a passion for gaming, mental and bodily labor, a residence in a marshy situation, or in a chamber that is not properly ventilated. If the cure is to be perfected as speedily as possible, we must avoid all these excitants"* (p. 281). And of course they must be avoided just as scrupulously in the "proving" as in the "cure," that the "totality of the symptoms" produced by the medicine under trial may be as unmixed as possible with the effects of other agents.

Hahnemann's statement of the mode of proceeding in the provings, is far from being clear and definite,

* The extreme caution sometimes practised by Homœopathists is very laughable. A gentleman had a camphorated preparation applied to his limb which he had injured. On going home, his wife, who was a thorough Homœopathist, made him go into the basement, and stay there day and night for three or four days, lest the smell of the camphor should interfere with the recovery of her children, who were sick in the nursery above, under the care of a Homœopathic physician. And ventilation, fumigation, and purification were all put in requisition, to prevent even an infinitesimal quantity of the camphor from ascending to the nursery, and neutralizing the infinitesimals administered to the dear little ones. There was ample compensation for the pain of the separation. The Homœopathic *cordon sanitaire* was effectual—the children recovered.

although in some respects he is quite particular and circumstantial. He does not tell us when we must begin to note down the symptoms; neither does he inform us whether they are to be noted down only upon the days when the medicine is taken, or whether the medicine is to be laid aside when the system is fully under its influence, and then the observation of the symptoms is to be continued so long as that influence lasts. We suppose that the latter is the course which he intends should be pursued, as he has marked down with great precision the duration of the effects of each remedy.

If the restrictions above named be faithfully observed, the subject of the experiment is to be considered as wholly under the influence of the medicine. Hahnemann (p. 210) holds upon this point the following very explicit language: "Provided all the conditions before stated be complied with, the symptoms, modifications, and changes of the health that are visible during the action of the medicine, *depend upon that substance alone*, and ought to be noted down as properly belonging to it." The medicine, though it be an infinitesimal portion of charcoal or common salt, or oyster-shell, is the presiding genius of the scene; it has control over the whole man, not only physically, but morally and intellectually also. Not only all bodily sensations, but all states of mind and heart, are to be noted down as the effects of the infinitesimal. The length of time that this is to be done depends upon the "duration of effects" of the medicine. In some cases this period is rather long. In the case of nux vomica, three or four weeks; sepia, seven weeks; oyster-shell, fifty days; sulphur, fifty days, etc. In such cases the records must be somewhat voluminous, and must require the patience of a stout believer to make them out.

Though the subject of the experiment is under the supreme control of the medicine, its action is somewhat *modified* by other agencies. And Hahnemann gives particular directions in regard to observing the circumstances which do thus modify it. For example, he says that in order to discover what is peculiar and characteristic in each symptom, the observer "should place himself successively in various postures, and observe the changes that ensue. Thus he will be enabled to examine whether the motion communicated to the suffering parts by walking up and down the chamber, or in the open air, seated or lying down, has the effect of augmenting, diminishing, or dissipating the symptom, and if it returns or not upon resuming the original position. He will also perceive whether it changes when he eats or drinks, when he speaks, coughs, or sneezes, or in producing any action of the body whatsoever. He must also observe at what hour of the day or night the symptom more particularly manifests itself."

I wish to have my readers understand and appreciate fully the mode of conducting the provings, and I shall therefore give a faithful representation of it. Suppose, then, that a person intends to prove upon himself the effects of some medicine. He studies carefully the directions of Hahnemann, that he may not spoil his experiment by any error of diet and regimen. He determines to abstain from coffee, tea, spices, seasoned viands, old cheese, pork, goose, duck, etc., and he gives the cook directions accordingly. He corks his wife's Cologne bottle tightly, and enjoins it upon her to remember that it must not be opened, and her perfume bag he locks up in a bureau in an unoccupied and distant chamber. All this being attended to, he composes his mind to an even state, and now he is prepared to swallow the potentized infinitesimal, and observe and record its effects.

Let us see how he makes his observations. After finishing his dinner he finds that he has not eaten as much as usual, and that his bread has remained by his plate untouched, and then he has not afterwards any desire for his customary cigar. He puts down, therefore—*Loss of appetite, chiefly for bread and tobacco-smoking*. In driving some nails into a box he is obliged to stoop, and when he raises himself up, he finds his head feels heavy and painful. He notes down—*after stooping some time sense of painful weight about the head upon resuming the erect posture.* On going out to see a friend he feels some stitches in one of his ankles as he steps *out* of his door, but does not feel them when he steps *into* his friend's door. He puts down—*stitches in the ankle when stepping out.* If on conversing with his friend, he finds himself more inclined to laugh than usual, he jots down—*inclination to laugh.* Or, if in some discussion with him he finds himself fretted with his friend's arguments, but anon disposed to be jocose and light-hearted, his record is—*alternation of fretfulness and hilarity.* In the evening he joins his wife in some fine crewel work, and he perceives that his hands tremble. He notes down—*tremor of the hands when occupied with fine small work.* He proposes a game at backgammon, but immediately remembers that " a passion for gaming" is one of the things to be avoided during a proving, and gives it up as a true devotee of the science should. He chances as he sits to scratch the sole of his foot, and thereupon there comes on a tickling there which provokes him very much, but at the same time is in some sense pleasurable. This symptom belongs to the " totalities," and he puts it down very circumstantially thus—a *voluptuous tickling on the sole of the foot after scratching a little, making a man almost mad.* In the night he has pains here and there, and his kind wife applies a poultice to some spot peculiarly painful, which relieves him. He notes down—*pains mitigated by warm cataplasms.* In the morning he hawks up some phlegm. He makes note of this—*phlegm is hawked out in the morning.* But he remembers that he has hawked a little at other times, and, as he wishes to be minutely accurate in his record of his totalities, he alters the record by inserting the word *chiefly* between *out* and *in.* In brushing his teeth he inadvertently uses his toothpowder, and this being " medicinal" in its character, and being therefore among the things prohibited, he supposes puts an end to the present "proving."

This may strike my readers as being a gross caricature of the Homœopathic provings. But it is in truth a fair representation. The notes made by my imaginary observer are *actual quotations from Homœopathic records of provings;* and all that I have imagined is the manner in which the observations were made upon which the notes were based. And the notes which I have thus quoted are by no means rare specimens of folly, obtained by diligent search through numerous tomes of Homœopathic wisdom. Such notes can be found in abundance on every page of Jahr's Manual, or of Hahnemann's six volumes of Materia Medica Pura.

Many such provings as I have depicted are made by many different persons, and then the records of them are collected and arranged. But the arrangement is very loose—there is no comparing or sifting; or if there be any, I see no evidences of it. The "totality," when fully made out from all the "provers," is, especially in the case of those remedies which are most commonly used, an endless farrago not only of ridiculous trivialities, but also of details of suffering, both bodily and mental, of the most horrid character. The tragic and the comic are mingled together in them after the most grotesque fashion.

That the reader may see that I do not at all overstate the matter, I introduce here a part of one of these compilations of provings. The article is sulphur. I give it exactly as it stands in Jahr's Manual. Why portions are placed in italics, neither the author nor the editor (Constantine Hering) is pleased to inform us.

"*Predominant Effects.*—Drawing, *rending and stinging* in the limbs, chiefly *the joints, with stiffness*, and intolerably increased pains under feather beds; wrenching pains; straining in the limbs as from decurtation (shortening or cutting short, *Webster*) of the tendons; spasm and crooking of the limbs; *arthritic swelling of the joints* with heat; pale, tense, hot, hard tumefactions; varices; *inflammation, swelling, suffocation and induration of the glands; scrofulous and rachitic complaints;* pains in the bones, as if the flesh were loosened from them; inflammation and swelling of the bones; incurvation of bones; *Caries* (bones both bent and mortified by sulphur, and that too in an infinitesimal dose!); *disorders from the misuse of cinchora and mercury; hysteric and hypochondriac complaints of various kinds;* chlorotic and icteric affections; gastric and bilious complaints; inflammations, *dropsical affections*, and suppurations of internal organs: *paralytic affections*; tingling in the limbs; *disposition to numbness*; easily injured in lifting; twitching of the muscles; *fainting fits and spasms*, also hysteric; single jerks in the limbs when sitting or lying; *epileptic paroxysms*, with a sensation proceeding from the back or arms, as if a mouse were running there. Tremor of the limbs. *The most complaints originate only when at rest*, and disappear by motion of the part affected, or by walking. *Pains appear or are increased at night.* The pains are exacerbated by the cold and relieved by warmth. *The patient feels worst in a standing posture.*

General restlessness in the body, which does not allow of sitting long, with an urgent disposition to stretch and draw up the limbs. *Strong agitation of the blood*, also after drinking beer (not I suppose after drinking anything else, wine, brandy, &c.); inward tremor; *fatigued by speaking;* languor in all the limbs disappearing by walking; infirm gait; *walking bent forward; great emaciation;* also with children; *great tenderness to the open air and wind, with a disposition to take cold; pains with the change of the weather; aversion to wash oneself.*

Itching in the skin, worst *at night*, or in the morning *in bed*, frequently with a sensation of soreness, or heat, or biting, or bleeding of the scratched spot; *eruptions after vaccination;* chronic eruptions with a burning itching; *miliary eruptions*, with soreness of the skin; *scabies, with rash*; yellow or liver-colored spots on the skin; moles; suggillations (black and other marks) after an inconsiderable contusion; *herpes; erysipelatous inflammations* with throbbing and stinging; *chilblains*, itching in the warmth; *galling of the skin in children. Rhagades.* The skin difficult to heal; suppurations; fistulous ulcers; suppurating *cystic tumors;* furuncles; *ulcers*, with rending, stinging, and tension, *easily bleeding and discharging a fetid pus; panaritia* (whitlow); warts; hang-nails; *corns*, with pressing, stinging pains.

Invincible sleepiness in the daytime, chiefly in the afternoon, and in the evening. *Late sleep in the evening* in bed; *nocturnal sleeplessness*, with restlessness and tingling of the limbs; too slight sleep; profound lethargic slumber in the morning; inability to sleep in any other way than in a supine or half sitting posture; *delirious, anxious, restless dreams, with fright in sleep* and fear when awaking; moaning, snoring, *talking* and *shrieking* in sleep; nocturnal wandering talk; *nightmare;* somnambulism; *shocks and jerks in the limbs in sleep.*

Chilliness, chills and sensation of coldness, without thirst; heat with much thirst; flushes of heat; quotidian fever, with heat and thirst after the chills; tertian fever, first coldness with thirst and drawing in the limbs, then chills, then heat without thirst, with a throbbing headache in the temples, (a very circumstantial record that—of course made by an experienced prover); chills with thirst, succeeded by heat; weakness, obstruction of the nose and scabs in the nose, with fever, (what kind of a relation weakness and a scabby nose have to each other, which should make it proper to put them together I cannot imagine); worm fever, (what, three fevers, tertian, and quotidian, and worm!); fever in the evening; nervous and hectic fevers, (more fevers still!); Perspiration in the morning or evening in bed; *Profuse per-*

spiration, in the daytime *when working*, and *at night in bed.*

Sadness and dejection; melancholy, with doubts about his soul's welfare; great inclination to weep, frequently alternating with laughing; inconsolableness, and reproaches of conscience about every action; *attacks of anxiety* in the evening; nocturnal fear of spectres; fearfulness, and *liability to be frightened;* restlessness and hastiness; caprice, moroseness, and ill humor; *irritability and fretfulness;* disinclination to labor.

Great weakness of memory; deliria and carphologia (delirious picking of the bed-clothes); mistaking one thing for another; *philosophical and religious reveries*, and fixed ideas; insanity, with imagination as if he were in possession of beautiful things, and in abundance of everything."

I have thus quoted about the fifth part of the totality of symptoms attributed by Jahr to sulphur. I will not tax the patience of the reader, or my own, with the rest. It is a very terrible totality. It differs somewhat, too, I may remark in passing, from the experience of my childhood, when every morning the teaspoonful of sulphur and molasses was swallowed as a preventive of a certain loathsome disease, whenever it was reputed to be prevalent. I felt nothing of all this totality, and my schoolmates did not; but we were mere boys, and none but men can be "provers," and Homœopathic men too.

But the totality of the effects of sulphur as it is, is

quite moderate compared with some of the other totalities. The symptoms recorded as produced by nux vomica, amounted a long time ago to about twelve hundred. How many the provers have added since, I know not. The totality of the effects of belladonna, as given in the "Materia Medica Pura," covers almost fifty octavo pages. And as early as 1838, Hering stated that the results of the provings had already filled more than fifteen octavo volumes.*

It is only by these provings, Hahnemann asserts, that we can acquire "a true Materia Medica." Each disease, you will observe, he regards as a mere group of symptoms, and asserts that there is in nature some

* In the brief notice which Dr. Joslin gives of his own conversion (as he styles it), he speaks of his recording the provings of medicines upon himself, and then comparing them with the "totalities." He says: "I took the third attenuation of a medicine, and, avoiding the study of its alleged symptoms as recorded in books, I made a record of all the new symptoms which I experienced. When this record was completed, I examined a printed list of symptoms, and was surprised to find a remarkable coincidence between them and those which I had experienced." He did the same with other medicines, as he says, with similar results. Each proving upon Dr. Joslin's person corresponded with the recorded totality of the medicine proved. He does not inform us, however, whether the "printed lists of symptoms" with which he compared his provings were the extensive totalities, or some of the limited ones. It would be interesting to examine Dr. Joslin's records of the provings which converted him. They would make probably a rich chapter in a history of conversions to Homœopathy, and I would suggest that they be given to the public just as they were noted down at the time. A full record of all the professor's sensations and moods of thought and feeling, while under the influence of an infinitesimal dose of charcoal or salt or oyster-shell, would be a curious contribution to the treasures of therapeutical science.

specific for every such group, which may be known by its producing a similar group of symptoms in the healthy. The "Materia Medica," therefore, according to his idea, cannot be complete till it embraces specifics for all possible groups or totalities of symptoms. And such a consummation as this Hahnemann confidently anticipated as being near at hand, and in view of it he exclaimed, "what cures shall we not be able to perform in the vast empire of disease, when numerous observers, upon whose accuracy and veracity we can rely, shall have contributed the result of their researches to enrich this "Materia Medica," the only one founded on fact. The art of curing will then approach to the same degree of certainty as the science of mathematics."*

The only remaining portion of Hahnemann's system, is his doctrine of the origin of chronic diseases, which is, that seven eighths of all these diseases come from psora, vulgarly called the itch. This fact, as he declares it unequivocally to be, he alleges that it cost him twelve years of research to establish. It is

* To aid in bringing about this consummation, Constantine Hering, that extraordinary physician, who, as the reader will recollect, has discovered that the small-pox "is so easily cured by one or a couple of doses of sulphur or rhus, that this disease should no longer excite any uneasiness," has proposed to his friend, A. Howard Okie, that a "Provers' Union" be formed in this country. Dr. Okie is delighted with the proposition, and thinks that the provers can do great things in making out the pathogenesis (these little dosers like big words) of the remedies submitted to trial. We shall expect large additions by this American "Provers' Union" to the totalities of the fifteen octavo volumes, if its members have any of the spirit of Yankee enterprise.

really only the old doctrine of humors, with a special, a sort of kingly prominence given to one of them, and that the most vulgar of the herd, despite of the pretensions of scrofula, erysipelas, and lordly gout. In truth, he degrades even these, which have so long held such proud sway in the "vast empire of disease," to a very menial rank, by announcing them to be *descendants of the itch itself.*

This psoric virus, which acts so large a part in disease,* is often very secret in its workings, and sometimes remains concealed in the system for a great length of time. It may produce "occasional outbreaks of disease," as Prof. Henderson expresses it; but, if the physician does not with his "anti-psorics" attack the constitutional taint, he will not rid his patient of the origin of all the evil, and, though he may cure him of his present obvious malady, there will be at some future time another outbreak. This may occur at a very distant period, even after the lapse of many years, the psoric virus having been latent all this time. "Hence," says Prof. Henderson (who, though he disavows anything like a full belief in the psoric doctrine, defends it in a

* It seems to be Hahnemann's idea that the itch has been working all manner of evil in the blood of man from the time of Adam, and yet Hahnemann was the first to discover it, for he says, "The modifications this miasm has undergone in its passage through millions of human constitutions, *during several hundred generations*, explain how it can assume so many forms." What a pity that the world had to wait six thousand years for the advent of the "Sage of Coethen"—the hero of anti-psoric medicine!

very labored manner, as not being "essentially unphilosophical"), "though *one chronic disease*, in the common acceptation of the term, may be perfectly and permanently removed, yet, if *another*, though totally different in its symptoms, should at any time subsequently appear, Hahnemann would have called it merely a different *form* of the same radical distemper, of the same chronic disease. So that if a man who once had some chronic disorder of his bowels, should, *twenty* years after it was removed, become affected with palsy, in Hahnemann's opinion it would have been the old disease recurring in a new form, either because the constitutional psora had not been cured along with the former illness, or because the taint had been contracted anew."

Dr. Wesselhoeft, in his reply to Dr. Holmes, says that Hahnemann did not assert that seven eighths of all chronic diseases come from the itch, "but that the Allopathic method of treating it made it a source of so great a part of the chronic diseases of our race." If this be so, what an untoward alliance this of Allopathy to itch, and what a numerous and motley progeny has it produced! Let, then, the alliance at once be annulled, and attack the psoric virus henceforth with the infinitesimal doses of Homœopathia, and thus let mankind be delivered from the multitude of chronic diseases that affect them. What a deliverance! Seven eighths of all the consumption, scrofula, insanity, idiocy, epilepsy, cancer, gout, dropsy, etc., etc., banished from the world! Why, it would introduce a physical millenium. Jenner's discovery is as nothing to it ; and Hahnemann is the great benefactor of the race !

Such is as plain a statement as I am able to make of the chief doctrines of Hahnemann. Before proceeding to an examination of them, I will state very briefly the points on which Homœopathists agree, and those on which they disagree, so far as I understand their meaning.

All of them believe in the great central doctrine of his system, *similia similibus curantur.* Most of them agree with him that it is the *sole* law of therapeutics, and, though none, so far as I know, plainly disavow this, yet there are some who practically, at least, admit the existence of other laws.

All agree in the efficacy of the infinitesimal doses. None, so far as I know, deny this, though some give medicines in doses of every variety, from the higher attenuations of Homœopathy up to the most *heroic* doses of Allopathy. Some differ from Hahnemann in their explanation of the mode in which the infinitesimals acquire their efficacy ; but this is a mere theoretical difference, and, therefore, is of no practical importance. Some, too, disavow his ridiculous idea of the importance of the number of shakes employed in the preparation of medicines ; but it is very far from being discarded by Homœopathists as a body.*

* In the first number of the "North American Homœopathic Journal," a periodical recently established in New York, and edited by Drs. Hering, Marcy, and Metcalf, one of the editors in commenting upon

All agree as to the mode of conducting the provings. Now and then one, like Prof. Henderson, when rallied on the subject, will grant that Hahnemann was a little too minute, and "did err in recording trivial occurrences." Still there is no plain and open avowal of any disagreement with him on this point on the part of any author which I have consulted, and the books of Hahnemann and others, which are filled *ad nauseam* with these "trivial occurrences," are the standard works among Homœopathists to this day. Not a hint has been made in regard to an expurgated edition of any of them. If it should be attempted by any modernized Homœopathist, he would be puzzled to know where to begin or where to end.

The psoric theory is far from being discarded by Hahnemann's disciples of the present day; and, though few of them do more than apologize for it, as Henderson does, yet most of them are inclined, with

"Jenichen's High Potencies," says, "Every one who prefers to make high potencies in his own way, may do it, but ought not to forget that Jenichen's preparations cannot easily be equalled, his last potence of arsenicum having received *one and a half million* of the most powerful shakings, counting only such as produced *a metallic ringing sound* of the glass bottle. Others may wait until the thing is accomplished by machinery, but they ought never to expect anything cheaper." This outstrips Hahnemann altogether. He never dreamed of one and a half million of shakes, and the test of the efficacy of a shake in dynamizing medicines being in its "metallic ringing sound," is altogether a new idea. The editor does not inform us whether the shakes were all of the true Hahnemannic character, with "a powerful shake of the arm *descending*," but I presume Jenichen took care to be orthodox on that point.

him, to talk of "anti-psorics" as "the most useful of the Homœopathic means" in treating chronic diseases, showing that they more than half believe the doctrine to be true. Dr. Holmes says of this doctrine playfully, but very truthfully, "I will not meddle with this excrescence, which, though often used in time of peace, would be dropped, like the limb of a shell-fish, the moment it was assailed."

CHAPTER III.

EXAMINATION OF THE DOCTRINES OF HOMŒOPATHY.

I PROCEED now to an examination of the doctrines of Homœopathy, and of its mode of practice. In doing this, I shall keep in mind the differences between Homœopathists, to which I referred in the conclusion of the last chapter, and shall have occasion to notice them in the course of discussion.

The principle expressed by the Latin phrase, *similia similibus curantur*, is declared by Hahnemann to be the "*sole* law of therapeutics." He asserts most explicitly, that all cures which have ever taken place, have been effected alone by this principle, whether they have resulted from the influence of medicine or the efforts of nature. He does not deny that physicians before him did sometimes cure disease; but he says that they did it ignorantly, and that the principle upon which they did it was undiscovered till his

In order to establish this doctrine as the *sole* law of cure, it must be proved beyond a question that cures are never effected under any other law. There must be no exceptions. If there be apparent exceptions, they must be shown to be only apparent—they must be proved to be consistent with the law. Till this is done—till all known cures can be demonstrated to be consistent with this law, there is no proof that there may not be other laws or principles by which cures are effected. And farther. If cures are made beyond a question by remedies acting on other principles, then the proof is absolute that this is not the *sole* law, though it may be one of the laws of cure.

Let us examine this point with some particularity.

If the doctrine, *similia similibus curantur* be the *sole* law of Therapeutics, the totality of effects produced by any article in the healthy, should be a sure indication that this article will relieve a similar set of symptoms whenever they appear in the sick. This should be found to be the fact *invariably* by experience. For example: opium produces in the healthy a state of insensibility and somnolency, and ipecac produces nausea and vomiting. Therefore, if the Homœopathic law be the *sole* law of cure, opium should invariably relieve insensibility and somnolency in the sick, and ipecac should invariably relieve nausea and vomiting. It matters not that they *sometimes* do this in some peculiar cases: to prove the law to be the *sole* law, they should *always* do it. It is upon these occasional peculiar cases that Homœopathists rely to show that these remedies act in consistency with their *sole* law of cure. The sophistry of such an argument, as the reader sees, is not only shallow, but contemptibly so.

Under this head I may also remark, that if *similia similibus curantur* be the *sole* law of cure, then a remedy should never produce in the sick effects similar to those which it produces in the healthy. For example. Opium ought never to produce somnolency in those who are wakeful from the influence of disease. So, also, it should never increase a somnolency already existing, but should always lessen it. This is so obvious that I need not dwell upon it.

Again. I take now the converse of the first proposition. If the Homœopathic law, be the *sole* law of cure, then, if any remedy cure a disease, or in other words remove any group of symptoms in the sick, it should be found invariably to produce a similar group of symptoms when applied to the healthy. Thus, if bleeding or blistering or both together have cured pleurisy (as experience has proved abundantly, whatever Homœopathists may say to the contrary), then bleeding and blistering should each, or together, produce symptoms resembling pleurisy in the healthy. Whether bleeding is apt to do this, any "prover" may discover, by inquiring of those who were wont to be bled regularly every spring, with the idea that it prevented sickness. He need not be under the necessity of "proving" it upon himself.

But lest the Homœopathist should not be satisfied

with this allopathic illustration, I will take one from Homœopathy also. Hahnemann and his followers assert most stoutly that camphor removes the totality of symptoms called cholera. If this be so, then, according to the *sole* law, we should find that camphor always produced in the healthy a totality of symptoms resembling this disease. Does it do this? Not at all. The effects of camphor upon the healthy are very far from being the "image of the disease" termed cholera. To make out these two totalities to be alike would tax one's credulity as much as it would to believe that a cow and an elephant bear a strong resemblance to each other. The effects of a hundred other substances resemble cholera quite as much as do those of camphor.

Again. If *similia similibus curantur* be the *sole* law under which cures are effected, then we should be able to prove, either that the vital powers are never competent to cure disease alone and unassisted by remedies, or, that they do it in conformity with the Homœopathic law. Hahnemann accepts the first horn of the dilemma; and expressly asserts that the cures alleged to be effected by the *vis medicatrix naturæ* are not cures. He has but a poor opinion of the efforts of the "unintelligent vital powers," and quarrels with "the vulgar practice" for its imitation of nature's bungling operations.

Now there is no fact more thoroughly established, both by common and professional observation, than that the curative tendency in the system is compe tent to cure a large proportion of the attacks of disease without the assistance of any remedy. This is certainly true of the numberless trivial ailments, slight colds, temporary headaches, etc., which so often get well without medicine, and alike with or without its shadow, the Homœopathic globule. Perhaps, however, the Homœopathist would claim that these are not really diseases, although each case manifestly presents its group, its "totality of symptoms." I remark again then, that what I have said of the curative tendency of nature is certainly true of all mild cases of what are termed self-limited diseases—those which have a certain defined set of processes to go through, such as measles, small-pox, etc. When these maladies have finished their course, the vital powers restore the healthy condition of the system, removing all the consequences of the disease. The same is true too of other diseases. In all mild cases, with proper diet and regimen, the vital powers are able to cure them. And in the practice of every judicious physician, a large share of the medication employed aims at assisting the curative tendency of nature, and removing obstacles out of its way, so that its action may be free and undisturbed.

As then the *vis medicatrix naturæ* effects cures, it has its principles upon which it does this—in other words, it has its laws of cure. The Homœopathic law of cure then is not the *sole* law.

But I go farther than this. Not only is it untrue that *similia similibus curantur* is the *sole* law of therapeutics, but there is no proof that it is even one among the many laws of cure which are employed in the removal of disease. Future observation *may* establish it as one of these laws, but Homœopathic observation has not done it.

Law is a word of high import in science. It means something more than a theory or hypothesis. Mere theory proves nothing. It may make a show of probability. That is, one theory or hypothetical explanation may be more probable than another. It may suggest, too, observation which may result in the discovery of a law. But in itself it has none of the attributes of a law in the proper meaning of that word. Nothing is worthy of being called a law but *a principle established upon good and substantial proofs.*

I am satisfied upon the showing of Homœopathists themselves, and I trust that I shall satisfy my readers also, that the doctrine, *similia similibus curantur,* is not one of the established laws of therapeutics; and not only so, but that as a theory it is exceedingly improbable. Almost all the facts to which Homœopathists appeal for the support of this doctrine, not only fail altogether to be explained by it, but they have a satisfactory explanation on other principles. And the remainder of these facts have as yet had none but a hypothetical explanation, and therefore it involves a mere estimate of probabilities to choose between a Homœopathic explanation, and that which may be based upon some other hypothesis. In deciding any question in science, such unexplained facts are of course not to be relied upon, however much they may be prized by the mere theorizer; and our reliance must be upon facts which in the present state of our knowledge we are able to explain.

Let us then examine some of the principal facts which Hahnemann and others adduce in support of the central doctrine of his system.

One of the facts greatly relied upon by Homœopathists, and very frequently quoted, is thus rather awkwardly announced by Hahnemann in his Organon, (p. 95.) "Frozen sour crout is frequently applied to a limb that is recently frozen, or sometimes it is rubbed with snow."

The idea of Homœopathists seems to be that a limb is frozen by cold as a positive agent, and that the cold united with water making it snow, or with the sourcrout, is only *similar* to cold united with air, and not the same thing. It is only upon such an unphilosophical, may I not say ridiculous, idea, that the fact referred to can be tortured into an illustration of the doctrine, *similia similibus curantur.*

But how is a limb frozen? Simply by the abstraction of heat. And how is it restored to its natural state? By a restoration of its heat; in other words, by the communication of heat to it. Whatever may be the applications, it is the heat in them that restores the limb. This can be done, either rapidly by warm water or warm air, or slowly by cold (that is, less warm) applications, in the shape of cold water, or snow, or "frozen sour-crout," it matters not which. And it has been found by experience that it is much better to restore the limb slowly, than it is to do it rapidly. This is the reason, and the only one, why we should not make warm but cold (less warm) applications to a frozen limb. The schoolboy recognizes the same principle when he warms his almost frozen fingers gradually, and thus avoids the aching which he knows by bitter experience follows too sudden a transition from cold to warmth He does it in a *cooler* air than he would do it in if he stood directly before the fire. In this case air, and not water, is the *medium* by which the heat is applied—this is the only point of difference between it and the case of the frozen limb restored by the snow or cold water.

To make the explanation still more clear, if necessary, observe the circumstances, under which a frozen limb is restored. When the snow, if that be the article used, is applied, it does not of itself restore the limb, but only moderates the process by which it is done. The warm air of the room restores it, and the snow prevents the air from doing it too rapidly. Snow would not restore it if the surrounding air were much below the freezing point, neither would cold water. The friction which is commonly used with the snow is not essential, but is a valuable auxiliary. It aids the restoration simply by exciting the nervous energy and the circulation of the part.

But Dr. Webelhœft asserts that the Esquimaux apply snow to frozen limbs in the cold air, and succeed in restoring them. This may be the case when the weather is not very severe, and when the limb is not badly frozen. The explanation is obvious. The enveloping snow acts as a non-conductor, preventing the air from abstracting the heat of the limb any farther, and the internal portion of the limb being still warm, and retaining its circulation, extends its heat outwardly, and in so gradual a way as to effect the restoration in the best manner. But this could not be done if the air were very cold, and if the limb were very thoroughly frozen; in that case, a resort to a warm apartment would be absolutely necessary.

The treatment of burns is often referred to as illustrating the operation of Hahnemann's law of cure.

It is the popular belief that a slight burn can be cured by holding the burnt part for a little time very near the fire. It is to be observed, however, that this expedient has the reputation of curing only in those cases which are so slight, that they would get well at any rate. But granting that heat does exert in such cases a curative influence, it certainly affords no proof of the truth of the doctrine *similia similibus curantur*. If heat will cure the effects of heat, it is not an example of *like* curing *like*, but of *same* curing *same*, which is quite another thing.*

* If this be the proper way to interpret and illustrate this law, hen opium should be the Homœopathic remedy for the effects of opium, calomel for the effects of calomel, etc. Indeed I once knew an experimenter in Homœopathy to administer a few drops of paregoric to relieve the effects of an overdose of laudanum. The overdose was

Besides if heat be the Homœopathic remedy for a burn—if it really have that peculiar "affinity" for it, which renders it a specific for that totality, then it should cure severe as well as mild cases. But this it is not pretended that it will do.

But it is said, that some of the applications which cure severe burns, such as alcohol and oil of turpentine, act upon the Homœopathic principle. If they do so, they ought to produce upon the skin in health effects similar to the "totality of symptoms" presented by a burn. Homœopathists may believe that they do, but it would be impossible for one not committed to Homœopathy to see anything but the very remotest resemblance between the stimulating effect of alcohol or turpentine applied to the skin, and that condition of things presented by a burn, especially if it be at all severe. The effect of mustard comes nearer to it, and therefore according to Hahnemann's rule, would be more Homœopathic to it; but who ever thought of treating a burn with mustard? Then too, there are other remedies successful in curing burns, which produce no perceptible effect upon a sound skin, such as sweet oil, a mixture of sweet oil and limewater, molasses, etc. No one will pretend that these articles produce effects which are the "image" of the disease or injury presented to us in the case of a burn.

not a large one—so the paregoric had the desired effect, just as heat cures burns that would get well if let alone.

It is to be further remarked in regard to the two cases to which I have referred, that they have no bearing upon the alleged efficacy of infinitesimal doses. It has never been pretended that an infinitesimal degree of heat will cure a burn, or an infinitesimal amount of snow or frozen sour crout will restore a frozen limb. Allopathic quantities are used, and dynamizing with "downward" shakes has never been suggested. Even the stimulating articles which are applied to burns, as alcohol and turpentine, are employed by the strictest of the sect in the "coarser" form, instead of a potentized dilution.

In the introduction to Hahneman's Organon there are more than fifty pages of what he terms "examples of Homœopathic cures performed unintentionally by physicians of the old school of medicine." The reasoning which appropriates these cases as proofs of the truth of the doctrine, *similia similibus curantur*, is of the loosest character. I know not where I have seen the rules of evidence so entirely disregarded as they are throughout these fifty pages. Statements, allusions and bare hints, that have the faintest semblance of relevancy to the point at issue, are pressed into the service, and gravely paraded as undoubted proofs. If a remedy chance in any case to be the *antecedent* of a recovery, though there be not the slightest proof that it was the *cause*, it is eagerly taken by Hahnemann as proof of his doctrine, if the disease recovered from bear the remotest resemblance to any effect that the remedy was ever known or imagined to produce upon the system. And though Hahnemann, as the reader will recollect, lays great stress upon observing the group or *totality* of symptoms presented by a disease, and the similar totality of effects of the remedy which cures it, yet in this incongruous detail in the Organon, he constantly bases his conclusions upon single symptoms, or upon groups so small, that they cannot with any propriety be called totalities. Some of his conclusions also are drawn from mere idiosyncrasies. Though it is obvious that no inferences can properly be made in regard to the ordinary effects of medicines, from any effects resulting from individual peculiarity, yet Hahnemann does not hesitate to make such inferences when they will suit his purpose, being careful, however, to avoid them when they will not.

Such modes of reasoning are constantly leading Hahnemann into the grossest inconsistencies. I must be content, however, with giving a single example from this large collection of so-called experience. Satisfying himself, as he does, with such loose resemblances between diseases, and the effects of their remedies upon the healthy, he often makes the same remedy to be applicable to diseases of various and even opposite character. Thus he speaks of Belladonna as the cure for hydrophobia, different kinds of madness and melancholy, scarlet fever, and "amaurosis with colored spots before the eyes." And I will not tax the patience of the reader with the long list of maladies to which he says that opium has a Homœopathic affinity, and of which it is therefore the remedy. How it can cover so many and such different totalities is not easily comprehended.

But suppose that the doctrine *similia similibus curantur* is true, how then, let us inquire, ought we to conduct the provings of remedies upon the healthy?

There should be great care in the selection of the subjects of the experiments. They should be persons in perfect health, so that the effects of disease may not be intermixed in our records with the effects of the remedy.

We should be very careful to distinguish the effects of medicine from the effects of other causes operating upon the system—air, food, water, mental influences, electrical and other states, etc. And when any doubt exists, it should be solved by experiments upon various subjects. Many and very accurate experiments must be made, and results must be very judiciously and laboriously compared, before the totality of the effects of any remedy can be fully and correctly ascertained.

The size of the doses used in these provings is a matter of no small importance. The effects of different doses should be carefully noted, so that a comparison may be instituted between them. Especially should this be done if in one case an ordinary dose be used, and in another an infinitesimal one.

These rules cannot but commend themselves to

the common sense of my readers; and yet Homœopathic observation *tramples upon them all.*

The records of the provings show that Homœopathic provers are not particularly cautious in the selection of their subjects. Indeed, in one of their standard works, Jahr's Manual (as the translator informs us in the introduction), the effects of medicines upon the sick are indiscriminately mingled with their effects upon the healthy.

Again. No distinction is made between the effects of the remedy and the effects of other causes. The Homœopathic observer takes his subject, and, as he thinks, *insulates* him, by cutting off the use of a few articles, coffee, spices, perfumery, etc. He does indeed consider that other causes affect him, but only as modifying somewhat the influence of the remedy which is under trial. In his view the subject is about as thoroughly insulated for his experiment, as the subject of the electrician's experiments is when placed upon the insulating stool. He makes his record accordingly, putting down all phenomena, physical, mental, and moral, that he witnesses in him, as the effects of the medicine.

And it makes no difference whether the dose is large or small, or even infinitesimal. At least so we may justly infer from the summings up of the records of provings, and from the hints which we find in Homœopathic books on the subject. Hahnemann himself, the great exemplar, is very lax on this point. His first provings were made with the ordinary doses used by physicians. And while in his Organon, (p. 203), he states in the text that the doses to be used are the doses ordinarily used by practitioners, in a note at the bottom of the same page he says that recently he had "judged it more proper to administer only doses that are very weak and extenuated to a very high degree." It is rather singular that he should make this announcement in a note, and only incidentally. If he had from proper evidence come to this conclusion, and had at all appreciated the importance of it, he would have inserted it in the text, and would have given his reasons for it in full. But Hahnemann makes little note of the difference between ordinary doses and the infinitesimals, great as you have seen it to be, either in the provings or in the treatment of disease. And the same is true of all Homœopathists.

The insulation of the system, so coolly assumed as a fact by Homœopathists, impossible as it is in relation to ordinary doses, is obviously a still greater impossibility in relation to doses of an infinitesimal amount. It is, we may say, a *self-evident* impossibility on the face of it, that a man can be subjected to the supreme control of an infinitesimal quantity of common salt or chalk, and that this should produce all the bodily and mental phenomena which he exhibits for days and even weeks.

But even if it were possible that substances should be so excessively diluted as Homœopathists pretend, and that an infinitesimal dose of any substance thus diluted should exert some considerable influence upon the system, that influence would inevitably be neutralized by the world of influences coming upon it from other substances, as minutely divided and as thoroughly agitated in the moving elements around us. Every breeze would come to us charged with attenuations of endless variety gathered from far and near, and the water of which we drink would be impregnated with infinitesimal doses of the thousands of minerals and medicinal plants, which in the lapse of years have been laved in it by the side of lake, or sea, or river. The succussions and triturations of the constantly agitated wind and water would be quite as effectual in extenuating and potentizing the substances suspended in them, as the Homœopath's rubbing with the sugar of milk, or his *downward* shakes with the thirty phials. The world would be a great laboratory of Homœopathic remedies, and we should be subjected to an endless and confused variety of secret but all-pervading influences.

The extensive groups of effects contained in the recorded collections of provings, are nothing but confused medleys. And I can see no characteristics by which one medley can be distinguished from another. They are all very much alike, and each seems to be a collection of all varieties of phenomena and sensations that could possibly be imagined. How the Homœopathist can make any practical use of them, is beyond my power to divine. The comparison of such totalities (extending in some cases over forty closely printed pages) with the symptoms of diseases as witnessed in the sick room, appears to my Allopathic mind as rather a formidable work ; and I think the reader will not accuse me of any want of candor when I say, that I doubt whether any such comparison is ever faithfully made by Homœopathic physicians.

The mode of Hahnemann's provings, which I have developed in these pages, is universally received by Homœopathists. Professor Henderson does indeed allow, in speaking of the "exuberance of Hahnemann's details," that he "did err in recording trivial occurrences among the symptoms that followed the taking of the medicines." But he denies that "his error in the smallest degree affects the practical use of his provings." A strange assertion is this. All error does practical harm, and just in proportion to the amount of the error. If Hahnemann in his provings has recorded but few "trivial occurrences," as Dr. Henderson seems to think, then his error is small, and the "practical use of the provings" is but little impaired. But, if what is trivial and irrelevant vastly preponderates over what bears any relation to the remedy, then the provings are worthless in practice. And this is just the truth in regard to those provings which were made with the ordinary doses. Very nearly all the records of their effects are irrelevant, and what is relevant cannot be separated from the mass of rubbish with which it is mingled. And the provings by infinitesimal doses have not even an infinitesimal amount of relevancy.

There are two errors in Homœopathic provings which are fatal to their practical usefulness; viz.: disregarding the difference between ordinary and infinitesimal doses, and assuming that all phenomena in the system come from the medicine under trial. And, even if it be true, as Homœopathists assert, that our knowledge of the influence of any medicine upon disease is to be derived from observation of its effects upon the healthy, this observation, in order to be of any practical value, must be conducted upon principles entirely different from those of the Homœopathic provings.

CHAPTER IV.

EXAMINATION OF THE DOCTRINES OF HOMŒOPATHY, CONTINUED.

THERE is much discrepancy between different leading Homœopathists in relation to the range of their doses; and not only so, but the practice of each one presents discrepancies, which show conclusively that Homœopathic observation of the influence of remedies upon disease is valueless. That the reader may see for himself that this is so, I will devote a little space to the examination of this point.

The doses administered in Homœopathic practice, especially at the present time, have an exceedingly wide range. Hahnemann himself, although he recommended the thirtieth dilution for common use, and asserted that even the smell of a globule containing the one thousandth part of a drop of this dilution, would, in some susceptible cases cure disease, did sometimes resort to even Allopathic doses, as for example in the treatment of cholera with camphor. Professor Henderson says that modern Homœopathists employ, especially in acute diseases, the lower attenuations for the most part, and sometimes even the original "mother tinctures." Laurie, of Edinburgh, says that he considers "the whole range from the first attenuation to the thirtieth, and even upwards, useful, according to the nature of the case." And Dr. Marcy of New York, (a prominent Homœopathist, I suppose, as he has published a system of theory and practice, and is one of the editors of a Homœopathic Journal), remarks—"We are constantly presented with well-authenticated cures by the undiluted tinctures and low dilutions, and have also as thoroughly understood and successfully practised the higher attenuations." His idea is, that there are "almost innumerable gradations of impressibility," requiring corresponding variations of doses; and this seems to be the idea of Homœopathists generally. The Homœopathic physician must, I think, have uncommon discrimination, if he can decide correctly in the case of each patient, to what point in this almost infinite scale of susceptibilities he belongs. And if he should chance to err, and give a dose of a low dilution, or of a "mother tincture" to a patient so susceptible, that he ought only to smell of a globule moistened with the thousandth part of a drop of the thirtieth dilution, the effect must be horribly destructive.

If medicines produce in infinitesimal doses such effects as are attributed to them, and if there be such wide differences in the susceptibility of the sick, it must be very important to fix upon exactly the right dose in each case. And if an infinitesimal dose of a medicine, carefully prepared with just the right amount of agitation and trituration, be appropriate to a case, then it would certainly be very injurious to the patient to give a million of such doses at once. Nothing can be more obvious than this; and yet Homœopathists do not appear to be aware of it, for in their dosing of the sick they jump about among the millionths, billionths, quadrillionths, and decillionths, with a sort of frisky freedom.

The range of doses in Allopathy is somewhat smaller than the range of doses in Homœopathic practice. For example, while the Allopathic physician calls the one sixth of a grain of tartar emetic a very small dose, and three grains (eighteen times that amount) a large one, the Homœopathic physician calls the decillionth of a grain a small dose, and a million, billion, quadrillion of such doses, what? Why, a small dose too. The arithmetic of Homœopathy seems to deprive those who venture its airy flights of all power of appreciating differences of quantity. Differences as wide as that between an atom and a world, they seem hardly to note or to know.

That my readers may see that I am not misrepresenting Homœopathic practice, I will refer them to some cases reported by Prof. Henderson. He is, perhaps, less adventurous than most Homœopathists in his leaps among the millions and trillions and decillions; and yet these cases show that it is not at all uncommon for him to change the medicine which he is giving in any case to the amount of six, twelve, even eighteen dilutions.

As one reads these reports of cases, the changes do not strike him as being so very great, because they are announced with such small figures. But if he undertake to estimate them, he finds that they are immense. Thus, when belladonna 12, is changed for belladonna 6, the alteration seems small, because the figures are so. But, in reality, a drop of belladonna 6 (the 6th dilution) contains, as I reckon it, just one hundred millions of millions more of the belladonna than a drop of the 12th dilution does. But he makes much greater leaps than this in his dosings. I could cite many examples from these cases, but one must suffice. In the case to which I refer (which the reader will find on page 42 of Henderson's Inquiry), the patient had taken, during the day, "bellad. 18," every hour, for three doses, and then every two hours, and at night it was changed for "bellad. 6"—a change, you observe, of twelve dilutions; and how many millions of millions that is, I will not stop to calculate. What a change of susceptibility must have occurred in only a few hours in that patient, to require such an enormous change in the amount of the dose! Or, perhaps, there was no such change of susceptibility; but the Professor found that the patient was not as susceptible as he first supposed, and that, on that account, he increased the dose. If so, I do not understand how he knew just what point to strike in this tremendous leap on the scale of doses.

That he did strike the right point, I suppose that he deemed to be certain; for he continued the medicine in the same dose the next day, and the day after the patient was well enough to go to his work.*

Absurd as this wide range of doses from the weaker to the stronger attenuations is, it is still more absurd when Homœopathists extend it still farther, and take in, as they now very generally do, the common forms of medicines. If, however, a mathematical law of the comparative effects of doses, which Hahnemann announces in his Organon as discovered by him, be really an established law, it at least lessens very materially the absurdity of this wide range of dosing. On the 297th page, he says: "The effects of a dose are by no means diminished in the same proportion as the quantity of the medicinal substance is attenuated." And in a note he states the law very definitely, thus: "Suppose that one drop of a mixture containing the tenth of a grain of any medicinal substance produces an effect= a; a drop of another mixtu recontaining merely an hundredth part of a grain of this same substance, will only produce an effect= $\frac{a}{2}$; if it contains a ten thousandth part of a grain, the effect will be= $\frac{a}{4}$; and if a millionth, it will be= $\frac{a}{8}$; and so on progressively. The effects of the remedy on the body

* Such cases show, either that it makes no difference what dilution is given, or that Homœopathic doctors have a wonderful tact at estimating degrees and changes of susceptibility, and that on a scale almost infinite. The latter horn of the dilemma will probably be accepted by most of them, as their modesty is rather Homœopathic in amount, and is apt to admit of assumptions of wisdom.

will merely be diminished about one half each time that the quantity is reduced nine tenths of what it was before." All this has a very scientific air, and looks like realizing the anticipation of Hahnemann, that the art of curing would at length "approach to the same degree of certainty as the science of mathematics." And if this doctrine be true, it is certainly a very important and wonderful discovery. But, formally and explicitly as it was announced, it never seemed to gain any currency among the followers of Hahnemann; and I believe that he himself has never even alluded to it in any other place in all his extensive works.

There is glaring inconsistency in the wide range of doses now so universally adopted by Homœopathists. If both ordinary doses and infinitesimal ones cure disease, they must obviously do it in different ways. The action of the potentized infinitesimal upon the system must be regulated by different principles from those which govern the action of the same article in its crude form. This truth is sometimes distinctly recognized by Hahnemann and other Homœopathic writers, in contrasting the effects of "coarse medicines" and attenuated ones. And yet they continually disregard it, both in their reasonings and in their practice.

Let me then illustrate this truth in a familiar manner You see a heavy weight raised by a rope. Suppose now that some one take from that rope a filament so small that it is invisible, and with this raises the same weight. We should say at once that the rope and the filament do not raise the weight upon the same principles—that some new power is given to the filament which is not possessed by the rope. 'True,' says the Homœopathist, 'that is clear enough; and we claim that a new power *is* given to medicine by trituration and attenuation!' Why then, I ask, do you not adhere to this view of the subject? You are nsistent with yourself. While you say that a w power is given to the infinitesimal which does not elong to the medicine in its crude state, and that by this power it cures disease; you at the same time claim, that the law, *similia similibus curantur*, is the principle on which both infinitesimals and crude medicines effect cures, which is as absurd as to say that the invisible filament raises the weight upon the same principle that the rope does.

But perhaps you will say that it is by some portion of the crude medicine, which by accident becomes attenuated, that the cure is effected, and that the same result would have been obtained if only an infinitesimal quantity of the same article had been used. If so, why use the mother tinctures and the crude medicines at all? And especially do I ask, why use the crude camphor in one of the most formidable of all diseases—the cholera; a practice which, so far as I know, is universal among Homœopathists?

The reader has observed that Hahnemann regards disease as a mere group of symptoms. He has nothing to do with their causes, and he uniformly speaks with contempt of all efforts on the part of physicians "to search the interior of the human economy." Upon this point he holds this language—"In what manner the vital principle produces morbid indications in the system, is to the physician a *useless question*, and will therefore, for ever remain unanswered. Only that which is necessary for him to know of the disease, and which is fully sufficient for the purposes of cure, has the Lord of Life rendered *evident to the senses.*" It is the external symptoms, therefore, that alone constitute in his view the disease, which he is to attack with his remedies.

And such are the views of Homœopathists generally. An abundance of evidence might be cited to prove this; but I will only quote as a specimen the language of Dr. Hering, one of the most prominent Homœopathists in this country. "The sole inquiry of the physician," says he, "is after the symptoms, because the symptoms alone determine his choice of a remedy; and upon the fullness or accuracy with which these are noticed, rests the entire management of the cure. All therefore depends upon the correct examination of the patient, and not upon any possible opinions concerning the *nature* and essence of the disease, nor upon learned views concerning its concealed *seat;* nothing indeed but the symptoms are to be accepted as the guide of the treatment, because in them no error is possible."

Very different from this are the views of Allopathic physicians. They find out, so far as they can, the *causes* of the symptoms, the *seat* and the nature of the disease, and for this purpose look at all the evidence which the present condition and the past history of the case furnish. We will take a very familiar example. If a patient have pain in the head, the rational physician considers it important to discover whether this symptom is produced by a disordered stomach, a determination of blood to the head, or some other cause; and applies his remedies accordingly. But the Homœopathist regards all such inquiries as "*useless questions*," and aims his remedies only at a group of symptoms, of which the pain in the head is one.

As Homœopathists look only at the symptoms which are "evident to the senses" as their guide in the treatment of disease, a knowledge of "the interior of the human economy," however interesting it may be to the curious mind, is of no manner of advantage to them. *They therefore, as a body, wholly neglect the study of anatomy, physiology and pathology.* These have no place in the science of their therapeutics. Some affect to deny this charge; but it is useless. The evidence of its truth is to be found on almost every page of standard writers on Homœopathy. The neglect of these departments of medical science, being the legitimate result of their doctrine, is everywhere palpably manifest.

Homœopathists attempt to support their doctrines by a great variety of illustrations, all of which are grossly fallacious. The fallacy of a few of them, I propose now to point out to the reader.

Many illustrations are drawn by Homœopathists from the effects of medicines in ordinary doses, well-pulverised or diluted. They would have us admit that, because some grains of a remedy will produce more effect when thus prepared than when it is given in a crude unprepared state in a large amount, therefore a single grain of it diffused through a liquid more in bulk than the whole world, or even many worlds, will give to each drop a peculiar medicinal power—a conclusion which is altogether too great a leap for common minds, and is within the capabilities only of such minds as have been "spiritualized" and "dynamized" by the etherealizing processes of Homœopathic belief.

The fallacy of the illustration from vaccination so often used by Homœopathists is of a similar character. Here an effect which pervades the whole system, it is true, is produced by a very small quantity of matter. But how small? Is it infinitesimal? Certainly not. Let the Homœopathist, instead of vaccinating some fifty or an hundred persons with a grain of the virus, make a solution of it so weak, that if a whole grain were used it would be diffused through whole oceans of water, and then let him vaccinate with this solution, and if he succeed in producing the vaccine vesicle, I will grant that his illustration would have some show of reason. But even then it would be in fact materially defective. For while the vaccine virus has the power of reproducing itself, and *thus* spreads from the mere point where it is introduced and affects the whole system, the infinitesimal globule has no such power, and if it produce any effect, must do it in altogether a different manner.

The same fallacy is seen in the illustrations which are drawn from the extreme divisibility of matter. A single specimen will be sufficient to exhibit the fallacy of all these illustrations.

Dr. Stratten, in his Preface to Hahnemann's Organon, in alluding to the scepticism of many in regard to the efficiency of infinitesimal doses, relates an experiment which he says "may serve to explain the degree of dilution substances are capable of. One grain of nitrate of silver was dissolved in fifteen hundred and sixty grains of distilled water, to which were added two grains of muriatic acid—a gray precipitate of chloride of silver was evident in every part of the liquor."

Dr. Stratten would have us believe, that because the grain of nitrate of silver diffused in fifteen hundred and sixty grains of water, could be visibly detected by a chemical test, therefore a grain of it, diffused through more water than is contained in all the rivers, and lakes, and seas, and oceans on the earth, would impart to every drop of it a medicinal power, that would produce manifest effects upon the system, and be effectual in removing disease. Like other Homœopathists, Dr. Stratten is somewhat careless as to relative quantities. If he should infer that because a rock or an elephant can crush a man, therefore a pebble or a flea can do the same, this inference, absurd as it is, would be nothing like as absurd as the one which he makes in regard to his experiment; for there is vastly less difference between a rock and a pebble, and between an elephant and a flea, than there is between his solution of nitrate of silver and the higher attenuations of Hahnemann.

But the error of Dr. Stratten's inference is not one of quantity merely. The fact that a substance diffused very minutely in a liquid can be detected by a chemical test, does not bear in the least upon the question, whether an extremely small quantity of an article minutely divided can affect the human system and cure disease. The two results have no relation, and no inference can be drawn from the one in regard to the other. No relation exists between them, even if the attenuation to which the test is applied is as minute as that which is used as a medicine—much less when it is vastly less minute. As well might Dr. Stratten infer that, because he can distinctly see his cow at a mile's distance, therefore her bellowing can be heard at the distance of a thousand or even a million of miles, as that, because a grain of nitrate of silver diffused in fifteen hundred and sixty grains of water can be detected by a little muriatic acid, therefore a single drop of a solution of it millions of millions of times weaker than this can produce perceptible medicinal effects upon the human system. The want of relation between the results is as palpable in the one case as in the other.

Homœopathists often speak of the imponderable agents as illustrating the action of their attenuated medicines, just as if powers can be given to common matter by trituration and dilution similar to those which are possessed by light, electricity and heat. Joslin says—"The higher attenuations are, in one sense, imponderable agents. Their medicinal part has no appreciable weight. Like light, caloric and electricity, they possess great activity." And he asks, "Who can say that if ponderable matter were made sufficiently fine, it would not exhibit as astonishing powers as light, caloric, or electricity? Who can say that these imponderable agents do not derive their activity from that very circumstance?"

What a brilliant idea, that light and heat and electricity are only common matter attenuated to a high degree, deriving all their powers from mere comminution, as Joslin believes, or from the "downward shakes" of Hahnemann, given to it in the great refining laboratories of nature. It is with such views of the astonishing revelations to which Homœopathy is introducing us, that Joslin says—"It is the destiny of Homœopathia, not only to effect a glorious revolution in the art of healing, but to lead to new views of the constitution of matter. She is to become the handmaid of physical science, as well as the mistress of practical medicine." We are to hail "the sage of Coethen" not only as the "Newton of medicine," but as a second Newton in the wide kingdom of general science!

Dr. Joslin gives the following illustration of what he deems to be the difference between Allopathy and Homœopathy in practice—"Had it been customary with the older surgeons to extract splinters from the fingers by pounding them with a hammer, and some one had ultimately hit upon the expedient of doing it with a needle, should we not have heard a great outcry against the innovation? Says the old orthodox surgeon, 'This small-dose system has no efficiency. I have been pounding here for two hours, and the splinter has barely started. My instrument is efficient, as you have evidence in the bruises. Do you think to dislodge the splinter with your insignificant Homœopathic needle point? It is contrary to the experience of three thousand years; it is contrary to all analogy. I would as soon think of harnessing a musquito before my gig. I have deliberately adopted this maxim: to believe nothing which is incredible except on evidence which is overwhelming.' The surgeon of the new school replies—'Your instrument is ponderous and powerful, but not efficacious. Its force is worse than wasted on the living and distant parts. You might pound the patient to a jelly, before the splinter would come out. If you happen now and then to hit it, you are just as likely to drive it in. My instrument is small but effective. The whole secret consists in applying the force at the right point and in the right direction."

This is both amusing and plausible. But is it true? Look a little at the terms of the comparison, and see whether Dr. Joslin had a due regard to relative quantities in making them. If you call to mind the Homœopathic arithmetic developed in a former part of this essay, you will see that the difference between a hammer and such a needle as would be serviceable in getting out a splinter, is almost as nothing compared with that between an ordinary dose of medicine and an infinitesimal one. If the hammer is to be considered as representing an Allopathic dose, then a needle, not only invisible, but so small as to defy all calculation or conception, must represent the Homœopathic dose.* That such a needle can get out a splinter, is just about as "incredible" as that infinitesimal doses can cast out disease; and we should hardly be deemed unreasonable, if we refuse to believe it, "except on evidence which is overwhelming." Besides, if the hammer represent medicine in its ordinary dose, almost all Homœopathists sometimes, not to say often, use the hammer, and Hahnemann himself used it in preference to the needle in the case of the cholera-splinter.

Hahnemann, in his illustrations of his theory presses everything into service that has the merest

* The same criticism could be made upon nearly all Dr. Joslin's illustrations, as to his disregard of relative quantities. For example, he speaks of the "successed" preparations of Hahnemann having such curative power, that we can cure with them "the most violent disease in a *man* by a dose which would not harm a *mouse*"—he should have said a flea—nay more, an invisible mite.

shadow of analogy to his ruling idea. I will give a few examples from a note on the 117th page of the Organon.

"Physical and moral diseases," he says, "are cured in the same manner;" and of this truth he gives the following illustrations.

"Why does the brilliant planet Jupiter disappear in the twilight from the eyes of him who gazes at it? Because a similar but more potent power, the light of breaking day, then acts upon these organs." So then, the sight of the planet Jupiter is, in the view of this second Newton of physical science, a physical disease in the "eyes of him who gazes at it," and it is removed in accordance with *similia similibus curantur*, by "a similar but more potent power, the light of breaking day." The dose, however, in this case, is not an infinitesimal; but the greater the dose of light the more perfect the cure.

"With what are we in the habit of flattering the olfactory nerves when offended by disagreeable odors? With snuff, which affects the nose in a similar manner, but more powerfully." Will a sniff from a phial containing a globule impregnated with the thirtieth dilution do this, or is it the experience of the old ladies that a good round Allopathic dose is necessary?

"By what means does the soldier cunningly remove from the ears of the compassionate spectator the cries of him who runs the gauntlet? By the piercing tones of the fife coupled with the noise of the drum. By what means do they drown the distant roar of the enemy's cannon, which carries terror to the heart of the soldier? By the deep-mouthed clamor of the big drum." Here come the large doses again. But if Homœopathy apply to this case, the "big drum" is not needed, but the finest squeak of a mouse trod upon by a soldier, should suffice to cure the whole army of its fear of the enemy's cannon.

"In the same manner mourning and sadness are extinguished in the soul when the news reach us (even though they were false) of a still greater misfortune occurring to another." So then, in accordance with the *sole* law, all other sources of consolation, even those of religion, are useless; and when any one is afflicted, the only way to cure him of this "moral disease," is to tell him of some one who has it much worse than he has. In this case, too, it seems that an infinitesimal dose will not answer. If a man break his leg, it will not cure him of his "mourning and sadness" to tell him of some one that has hurt his little finger—a dose as large as two broken legs, or even a broken neck, will be required, especially if the patient is not very susceptible.*

* Though there may be in these cases of "moral disease," Dr. Marcy's "almost innumerable gradations of impressibility," they do not seem to admit of his infinitely wide range of doses. To be consistent with his Homœopathy, (and this is that of most of his sect,) while the stout imperturbable man, bowed down with "mourning and sadness" should require a truly Allopathic dose of others' woes to cure him; if the case, on the other hand, be that of a delicate hysterical lady, ever ready to feel and to weep, the story of some accident to a mosquito, a flea, or even a mite, poured into her ear in almost inaudible whispers,

Mr. Marmaduke Sampson, an English amateur Homœopathist, outstrips even the great exemplar in some of his moral illustrations. For example, he says—"The symptoms of mental excitement produced by ardent spirits, are in like manner most quickly and effectually overcome by means capable of producing symptoms of an analogous kind. A fright will do this, or any other sudden cause; and hence Cassio's immediate recovery from intoxication under Othello's reproof, is strictly in accordance with nature." Cassio's account of the matter, in reply to Iago's inquiry, "How came you thus recovered?" was, as the reader will recollect, "It hath pleased the devil, drunkenness, to give place to the devil, wrath." Though by a stretch of fancy we might make out some little resemblance between these two devils, there certainly is not enough in the "totality" of their characteristics to make one devil homœopathic to the other. A bucket of cold water would have been quite as effectual a cure for Cassio's intoxication as Othello's reproof was; and this remedy for such an excited inflammatory moral disease, is decidedly *Anti*-pathic, not Homœopathic in its character.

should suffice to relieve her. This infinitesimal dose of woe, should, by virtue of its "affinity" for the disease, go directly to it, as surely as the dynamized globule does, and any very large dose would "put in jeopardy the life of the patient," by introducing an "artificial disease" which the "vital force" would not be competent to remove. But whatever may be the experience of Homœopathists on this point, I have never heard of such a patient's being overwhelmed, or having her heart broken, by the bungling administration of too large a dose, too heavy a tale of others' sorrows.

But enough of these illustrations. I will not weary the reader with going through all even of the most common and prominent illustrations which we find in Homœopathic books, as substitutes for arguments and proofs. The totality of these fallacies is a large and incongruous totality.

The *inconsistencies* of Homœopathy are glaring and numerous. We find them alike in its statements, its reasonings, and its practice. I have exposed many of them incidentally in the course of my examination of this system ; but it may be well to notice some of the principal ones together, that the reader may see what a medley of inconsistencies this so called science presents.

The reason that attenuated medicines produce such a decided effect in the removal of disease is, according to Hahnemann and all Homœopathists, that the diseased parts are in a very susceptible state—implying, that if there were no such increased sensibility, the infinitesimal would not produce any effect, or at least an exceedingly slight one. Yet in the provings upon the healthy, in whom this reason for a decided influence from the infinitesimal does not exist, they record a large number of very decided effects from infinitesimals. To this they add another inconsistency still more gross and palpable. They record in their collections of provings indiscriminately, symptoms occurring under the use of both crude drugs and dynamized infinitesimals ; though they assert that the latter act upon the system by virtue of a new power given to them in their preparation, and of course cannot produce effects analogous to those of the former. And, to complete this jumble of inconsistencies, while they thus mingle together in these records the effects of crude and attenuated medicines, they explicitly assert, as an argument against the use of large doses, that the apparent effects of such doses are for the most part, sometimes entirely, the efforts of the system to resist and throw off the medicine, and that its legitimate effects can be ascertained only by administering it in small doses.

Again, in relation to doses. It is said that the amount of the dose must be proportioned to the degree of susceptibility in the sick; and some, perhaps we may say most Homœopathists, find such differences of susceptibility in their patients, that their range of doses takes in not only all the attenuations, but even the "mother tinctures" and crude drugs. Now the susceptibility is generally greater in acute than in chronic cases, and therefore, according to the rule, the higher attenuations should be particularly applicable to acute diseases. But no. They are used most in chronic cases, and in the acute the lower attenuations, and even medicines in their "coarse" form are employed.

Though Hahnemann was so exceedingly particular in "dynamizing" his infinitesimals, and so absolute and positive in rejecting the coarser forms of medicines, yet he prescribed camphor in the coarser form for so grave a disease as cholera. And his followers have universally adopted this practice, and reckon their greatest triumphs in the treatment of this disease with Allopathic doses. There is certainly an apparent inconsistency in this abandonment of infinitesimals in the treatment of cholera. Perhaps it can be shown to be only apparent and not real; but, so far as I know, no one has attempted to do this, and the most profound silence has been observed on this point by all Homœopathists, though the inconsistency has been pointed out to them again and again.

Great pains have been taken by Homœopathists to collect the totality of the effects of every medicine, and much stress is laid upon the importance of tracing, in each case, the relation between this totality and its counterpart, that is, the totality of symptoms belonging to the disease of which the medicine is the cure. Accordingly it is claimed, and if the premises be correct, the claim is a true one, that much study and skill are requisite in order to trace this relation faithfully, and that therefore, while Allopathy requires but little research, no one can be successful in Homœopathic practice unless he be a hard student and a skilful observer. But is this relation between the totalities really made the subject of much study by Homœopathic physicians? Do they make *any* use of the monstrous groups of symptoms recorded in Hahnemann's materia medica, in the investigation of cases as they occur in daily practice? There is no evidence that they do; and, on the other hand, there is much evidence that they do not. The records of cases which we find in their books and journals, instead of showing minute research, are ordinarily exceedingly jejune, compared with the totalities of the provings. In their reasonings too, the large totalities are forgotten, and inferences are made from very small groups of symptoms, or even from a single one. Totalities, it seems, like the doses, enlarge and contract to their convenience, ranging from a solitary symptom up to groups of a thousand or more, spread over forty or fifty pages. The boasted success of the lady Homœopathists, who practice with box and pamphlet, it may also be remarked, is hardly consistent with the alleged necessity of severe study and minute research in Homœopathic practice. To them this "difficult but beneficent art," as Hahnemann calls it, seems in some way to be made wonderfully easy.

Great pretensions to accuracy are made by Homœopathists; and yet you have seen not only how much they differ from each other in the range of their doses, but how extremely loose they all are in regard to the amounts of medicine they administer in different cases; and sometimes even in the same case. So loose are they in this respect, that the conclusion is forced upon us, that it makes no difference to them, or to the patient, whether the thirtieth dilution be given, or one which is millions upon millions of times stronger than this. Their palpable inconsistency on this practical point can be accounted for on no other supposition.

To trace out the totality of the inconsistencies of

the Homœopathic doctrine and practice would be an almost interminable task; and the group which I have presented of some of the most prominent of them, will suffice to convince the reader, that it is mockery to bestow the name of science upon such a mass of incongruities as are found in Homœopathy.

Such is the character of the system of medicine founded by Hahnemann. If I have represented it truthfully, *its great central doctrine, if true at all, applies only to a very small range of phenomena; its mode of observation is capable of establishng no facts, and it is therefore of no practical use; and the treatment of disease, based upon this mode of observation, must therefore be utterly absurd.*

CHAPTER V.

PRACTICAL EVIDENCES OF HOMŒOPATHY.

But it is said by the advocates of Homœopathy, that whatever may be thought of its doctrines, in practice it is successful; and therefore it must be true.

Here we come to the very citadel of Homœopathists. Whenever their doctrine is most clearly shown to be absurd, they retreat at once to the argument, of which every quack from time immemorial has been so fond. 'There are our cures—our facts,' say they. 'On *them*, after all, we rely for the proof of the truth of our doctrine.' The claims of Homœopathists on this point are exceedingly impudent. Joslin but echoes the general voice of his sect, when he says—"Hahnemann was the first who made well-ascertained facts the essential basis of the whole therapeutic fabric;" as if all physicians before him were a set of theorists and dreamers, and were no discoverers of facts. And he asserts it to be the grand peculiarity of Hahnemannism, that it relies upon facts, and facts alone. He ranks it in this respect with the Baconian philosophy, and even with Christianity itself. On this point he says—" Christianity was presented to the world in the shape of facts. It was a grand exhibition of the inductive method of philosophy. Now we may also claim for Homœopathy an inductive character, and for its believers a rational regard for the evidence of their senses." And again he says—" Such has been the course pursued by the disciples of Bacon, and also by the disciples of a still greater Master. These appealed to facts as the basis of their belief, and warned their brethren against the prevalent " philosophy," which was far from being inductive. The Greeks sought " after wisdom," after plausible hypotheses, and therefore rejected the facts and the true wisdom. The sophists, the self styled philosophers, held the same position as those medical sceptics of our day, who array *a priori* argument, barely plausible, against facts well attested."

Such being the claims of Homœopathists in regard to the practical proofs of the truth of their system, I wish the reader to examine with me candidly and faithfully the character of their boasted facts.

It is alleged in proof of the truth of Homœopathy by those who believe in it, that they have themselves witnessed cures performed by Homœopathic remedies. That they have seen persons restored to health while taking these remedies, I will allow ; but this by no means proves that the remedies cured them. Something more than the relation of antecedent and consequent is required to prove a real connection between the remedy and the recovery. The fallacious reasoning which is very prevalent on this point, both in the profession and in the community at large, is the great source of the delusion and quackery that abound in the world, and it has its full share of influence in maintaining the hold of Homœopathy upon the popular belief. I will therefore illustrate this point with some particularity.

In every case of disease there are many elements at work; and we accordingly see various actions mingled together in a manner more or less confused, viz,; actions strictly morbid in their character—actions dependent upon the natural course of the disease—restorative actions—those resulting from sympathy between the organ particularly diseased and other organs—and those which are produced by external agencies, some of which are known and others are unknown. All of these are to be taken into the account in estimating, in any case, the influence of remedies. With the observance of the utmost caution there is liability to mistake in our inferences on this point; and the liability is very great if the observer is incautious, and especially if he is wedded to any theory or system. And in the case of Homœopathy this liability is unusually great; because Homœopathic observation makes almost no allowance for the operation of the different elements to which I have referred, but shuts its eyes to the existence of nearly all of them, and with a wholesale credulity attributes nearly everything to the agency of its potentized infinitesimals.

Different degrees and kinds of proof are needed in different cases to establish a connection between the remedy and the recovery. As a general rule, it is true, that the more apt a disease is to end in recovery, the greater is the liability to mistake as to the influence of remedies. For example, in tetanus (lock-jaw), so apt is the disease to end in death, that if any particular remedy or course is followed by a recovery, there is strong presumptive proof that the remedy or course cured the disease; and but a few such cases would be required to establish its value in the treatment of this malady. In this case all the elements commonly work wrong, or at least fail to do good. If therefore any element which is added is followed by a recovery, even though it be tested upon only a few cases, we may safely conclude that the additional element is not only the antecedent, but the cause of the cure. But in a case where the elements work variously, well or ill, it is not so easy to discover the exact influence of the added element. For example, in such diseases as pneumonia and fever, in which the restorative agencies are prominent in the movements of the case, and are ordinarily competent to effect a recovery without the aid of art, it requires accurate and varied observation to determine the real influence of any remedy. Especially is this true in regard to those diseases which vary much in the different cases in their tendency to a recovery. Scarlet fever and cholera may be cited as examples. Accordingly a loose observation of these diseases in different localities and at different times has given to us a vast variety of remedies and modes of treatment, each demonstrated, as it is claimed, by experience to be preëminently successful.

The application of these principles is well illustrated in the cure and prevention of that dreadful disease, hydrophobia. So strong is the tendency of this malady to end in death, that but a small number of cases would be required to establish the value of any true remedy. But, on the other hand, a very large number of well-observed facts would be needed to prove any article to be a real preventive, because so few of those who are bitten by dogs supposed to be mad have the disease, whatever be the treatment. It is from a disregard of the principles which I have indicated that so many preventives of this malady have been successively adopted and discarded by the public. If there really be any preventive, there has as yet been no observation of such a character as could establish its claims.

Let the believer in Homœopathy apply these plain principles in his observation of disease, and he will find that much doubt will at once be thrown over the results which are claimed to be effected by the infinitesimal globules; and he will be convinced that an accurate sifting of evidence is necessary to determine whether any, and if any how many, of the apparent cures of Homœopathy are anything more than apparent.

But the advocate of Homœopathy will say that he does not judge from single cases; but that he has seen much of Homœopathic practice in his own and in other families, and compared it in relation to its results with Allopathic practice. But is he sure that his experience has been of such a range and of such a character, as to warrant his conclusions? I would suggest the propriety of a little caution on this point; for I have often known such conclusions, though very firmly adopted, to be given up from after experience, and similar conclusions to be as firmly adopted in their stead, in regard to some other mode of practice. Besides, the advocates of all the various systems of practice, and of all the numberless quack remedies, found their conclusions as to the success of their favorite remedy or system upon the same kind of experience. Each thinks all the rest to be mistaken, and perhaps pities their credulity, and dreams not that he commits an error precisely like theirs in his reliance upon the *post hoc propter hoc* mode of reasoning. The same is true to some extent also, of those physicians who have been the warm advocates of any one mode or system of practice to the exclusion of others. Each founds his preference upon experience—upon what he has seen of the results of different modes of practice. But all of these exclusive systems have, one after another, passed away; because a wider, more varied, and more prolonged experience, has shown the conclusions of their advocates to be false. All this ought surely to teach the Homœopathist some caution in making inferences from an experience of so narrow a range, as that which only a few families can furnish.

But it is said further, that many Homœopathic physicians once practised Allopathy; and that their testimony is very decided as to the comparative success of the two modes. Even allowing the conversion in every case to have been a rational one, produced by an honest and intelligent examination of evidence, and not one which resulted at all from pecuniary considerations, I think their testimony is not to be received implicitly, and without some questioning on our part. From what, I ask, have they been converted? From Allopathy, you say. But what is Allopathy? Is it one thing—one mode—one system? By no means. This term is applied to all kinds of practice pursued by all regular physicians. It is a very extended, and a very diversified combination. It includes much that is good, and much that is bad. And the practitioners of this Allopathy are, some of them, bad practitioners. Suppose now that the converts to Homœopathy are from this class, and not from among the judicious practitioners. If this be the case, then their testimony to the greater success of Homœopathic practice is good for nothing in regard to the question, whether a *judicious* Allopathy is less successful than Homœopathy. It only shows that Homœopathy is better than *bad* Allopathy. And this is undoubtedly true; *for doing nothing in the treatment of disease, is better than doing badly can be in any form.*

I wish not to speak harshly of Homœopathic physicians; but truth obliges me to say, that so far as I know, those regular physicians who have become Homœopathists, did not bear the character of judicious practitioners previous to their conversion. And they are doing less harm now with their sins of omission, than they would have done if they had continued their sins of commission in their undiscriminating over-dosing. Their testimony on that particular point can be taken; but when they testify in regard to that of which they have had no experience, a *judicious* Allopathy, their testimony is clearly not admissible.*

Besides, Homœopathy, that is, true, consistent Homœopathy, is not really put to a full test in the ordinary practice of its advocates. To make a fair trial of it, there should be a strict adherence to the principles of the system. There should be no mixing of

* Much boasting has been made by Homœopathists recently over the conversion of a French physician, M. Tessier, to the infinitesimal practice. Taking his own account of the matter, it is quite clear that his conversion is a very fortunate event for his patients. His was certainly *bad* Allopathy. He was a perfect Sangrado. How many times it was common for him to bleed in pneumonia, (the disease in regard to which he testifies,) he does not inform us; but he speaks, in his account of the experiments which led to his conversion, of his "diminishing the bleedings by one, by two, by three, by four," successively, introducing in place thereof the Homœopathic remedies. It is no wonder that he found Homœopathy more successful than *such* Allopathy as he practised. M. Tessier in his conversion ceased to exhaust and kill his patients by profuse bleeding; he thinks that he saved them by infinitesimal globules.

practice—no resorting, either openly or by stealth, to common doses, nor to other Allopathic measures, when the infinitesimals fail, or when the physician fears to trust them, on account of the violence of the disease. Now Homœopathy is ordinarily put to no such test as this. There is evidence in abundance that Homœopathists often resort to the Allopathic practice which they so much condemn.* They have always used

* Of the many facts in proof of this, which have come to my knowledge, I will mention but two.

A box, which was evidently the property of some Homœopathic doctor, was picked up in New York, and was put into the hands of Dr. James Stewart. It contains sixty-four phials. Most of these are filled with little sugar pellets, and are labelled in the usual Homœopathic style. There are some eight or ten, however, that are not thus labelled. These contain calomel, morphine, Tartar Emetic, &c., in the usual form and strength of Allopathists, the names being marked on the under side of the corks, so that they might be concealed from the eye of any over-curious patient who might look into the box. The design of all this is so obvious, that it needs no remark. The owner of the box has never claimed his property, although it has been very effectually advertised by being made the subject of an article in a New York Journal.

A gentleman who was suffering severely from neuralgia, was induced by his friend to dismiss his regular physician, and to place himself in the hands of a prominent Homœopathic doctor in one of our cities. As the opiates upon which he had relied to obtain relief to his pain were discontinued, his sufferings became intense. He insisted upon having something to relieve him; but the doctor refused, because he did not believe in palliatives, and wished, as he said, to strike at the root of the difficulty. On being told, however, by the patient, that he should go back to Allopathy, if he did not give him relief; he left three powders, which were "excessively bitter, more so," he says, "than anything I ever tasted." No relief came. The next day the doctor said—"the powders I left yesterday were not strong enough—*I will fix you to-day,*" and he left three more powders. After taking the last one, the patient soon became convulsed, then deranged, and he barely escaped death.

ordinary doses in some cases ; and now it has become so common to do so, that they are openly shifting their ground, and many, perhaps we may say most of them, allow of the use of all kinds of doses. Some, like Professor Henderson, admit in some cases even such Allopathic measures as bleeding. The result of all this is, that the artful Homœopathic physician is enabled to secure all the benefit which accrues from the popularity of the prevalent delusion, and at the same time escapes the sad results which would occasionally follow a strict adherence to the principles which he so stoutly, but so dishonestly advocates.

The ordinary testing of Homœopathy is deficient in still another respect. The Homœopathic physician, if he adhere with any degree of strictness to his infinitesimals, never has, at least for any length of time, a practice of such a character as the Allopathic physician has—viz. ; a steady family practice, remaining very much the same from year to year. His practice is more changeable than that of the Allopath. Though some families, in whose circle no untoward event has chanced to occur, may adhere to him steadily, he has

The medicine was undoubtedly *strychnine*. And this *enormous* over-dosing was done by a man who has been known to send corks from his phials to a patient to smell of to cure her disease.

It is often said by those who conclude to *try* Homœopathy, that it can at least do no harm. But to say nothing of the valuable time often lost in this miserable trifling, the patient knows not but that he may be *cheated* into dangerous medication, as was done in the case just cited, and in that of the Duke de Canizarro, who died a martyr to his confidence in Homœopathic honesty.

for the most part a very variable set of employers. He has, too, a much larger proportion of chronic cases than the Allopathic physician. People are not so ready to trust him in acute, as they are in chronic diseases. Now, to many of the chronic patients under his care, it would be injurious to take much medicine, and globules "potentized" by their imaginations, coupled with the confident promise of a certain, though gradual cure, are ordinarily the best medicines for them. Many of this class of patients are always getting better, but never get well ; and such, though certainly not very bright trophies of Homœopathy in the eyes of bystanders, are among the staunchest advocates of the system.* The facts above referred to, I may remark in passing, show why it is that Homœopathy is most rife in large communities, especially in cities. It cannot ordinarily live long in small places, because it cannot find there successive sets of believers, as it can in large communities.

The remarks which I have made in regard to the general character of the practice of Homœopathic physicians, are well illustrated by a detail of cases given by Professor Henderson. These cases are one hundred and twenty-two in number, taken from both private and dispensary practice. They occurred, as I see by the dates, during a period of eighteen months.

* A clerical friend who has seen much of Homœopathic practice says, that he never knew one of all the multitude of enthusiastic lady Homœopathists that was not always ailing and always taking pellets. This I suspect is true everywhere.

"The whole narrative of cases," he says, "is but the transcript of notes of general practice," and "will afford a tolerable specimen of what my own practice has presented me on the subject." He gives us to understand that he has made no selection from his cases suggested by the effects of treatment; but has presented all those of which he took notes at the time of their occurrence, with the exception of "cases so unimportant, that a detail of the speedily successful issue of them could not bear upon the question at issue, unless hundreds of them had been collected." He leaves out also, I find, cases of consumption and of fixed organic disease. "The cases recorded," Professor Henderson says, "constitute, I believe, scarcely a fifth of those which I have treated Homœopathically." The whole number thus treated by him was therefore about six hundred.

About three-fourths of the one hundred and twenty-two cases described in his narrative, are cases of *chronic* diseases. All cases of consumption and organic disease being excluded, this is a very large proportion of chronic cases of other kinds—vastly larger than would be found in any fair representation of the "general practice" of Allopathic physicians. Most of the thirty or thirty-five *acute* cases narrated by Dr. Henderson are really not at all severe, and, as Dr. Forbes says, "every physician of experience would have expected them to get well under any treatment." They are certainly so "unimportant" that his own rule should have excluded them. Of the remainder of the acute cases, two are cases of lung fever—a small number of patients with this disease, surely, in a practice including six hundred cases. And there are no cases of fever, pleurisy, acute inflammation of the bowels, colic, and many other diseases, which are met with so frequently by Allopathic physicians, and which would be recorded by them in a "transcript of notes of general practice." It is remarkable also that there are only five cases recorded of disease in very young children; and of these one is a case of chronic eruption, and another is one in which Allopathic treatment had been pursued, and death was at hand when Dr. Henderson was called, so that he only gave a little medicine in compliance with the importunities of the mother, and without any effect. So then, Dr. Henderson in his "Notes of a general practice," extending over a period of a year and a half, and embracing about six hundred cases, finds among the one hundred and twenty-two cases worthy of record only *three* cases of acute disease in young children which were important enough to be noted down. And yet, in the practice of every Allopathic physician, a very large proportion of his patients are young children; and if he were to note down, as Professor Henderson did, one of every five of his cases, in order to test the efficacy of any mode of practice in its general application, very many of his cases would be drawn from this class of patients.

If then Dr. Henderson has given in his narrative of cases a fair and candid representation of his practice as a Homœopathic physician, as I believe he has, at least, so far as it can be done by one who is committed to a " foregone conclusion," it is obvious that his practice embraces a much larger proportion both of mild cases, and of chronic ones, than that of most Allopathic physicians. And this is true of Homœopathists generally. It is evident, therefore, that Homœopathy is subjected to no such thorough testing in daily practice as Allopathy is. It does not ordinarily have to grapple with cases of every variety, and of every degree of severity. Indeed, it is very common for families, while they trust to Homœopathy in all mild cases, to reserve to themselves the right to fall back upon Allopathy, and even Allopathic physicians, whenever disease assumes at all a grave aspect. And I cannot forbear remarking here, that such families sometimes find to their sorrow that they have relied upon the tiny dosing too long. They forget that disease sometimes appears mild to the non-professional and unskilled observer, while it may be in reality of the gravest character. Some sad cases might be cited in illustration, but it is not necessary.

But again, it is said that statistics show very clearly that Homœopathic practice is much more successful than any form of Allopathic practice. But are these statistics, I ask, to be received as being of course correct and true? The value of statistics, and especially when they relate to therapeutics, depends upon the principles on which they are collected, and the mental and moral character of him who collects them. It is often said that "figures cannot lie;" but the annals both of quackery and of medicine show, that false statements can be made as easily in figures as they can be in words. Thorough, impartial observation is not a very common thing in medicine. That the observer may be impartial, he must not only have a strict veracity, but he must be bound to no theory nor system—he must be committed to no "foregone conclusion." This is especially true of therapeutical facts, because they are so multiform, and because as you have seen, they result from so many combined agencies. And for the same reasons *bare* statistics in therapeutics, even though they are collected in good faith, are of little value, although it is quite fashionable just now to rely upon them even among medical men. But if statistics are based upon a minute record of individual cases, and are gathered by competent and faithful observers, they are among the most valuable sources of knowledge in the treatment of disease.

If the statistics of Homœopathy be tested by the principles which I have indicated, they will be found wanting in those qualities which command our confidence. We will take for example its statistics of cholera. It was stated, after the first visitation of this disease in Europe, as the grand result of these statistics, that while the average mortality under the "regular" treatment was about forty-nine in one hundred, under Homœopathic treatment it was only about six in one hundred. This, you will observe, is an enormous difference. If the statement was really true, it is wonderful that the Homœopathic treatment of this disease has not been adopted by this time all over the world. *It would have been, if the statement had been believed.* But it has not been believed.

Let us see now whether physicians and the community generally have withheld their belief for good reasons; or, as has been asserted by Homœopathists, from a wilful and wicked obstinacy. These statistics, it is to be observed, are, for the most part at least, *bare* statistics, unaccompanied with any details of cases. They are made by men who are committed to a theory and to a system of practice, and who show, by their "provings" and their records of cases, that they cannot be relied upon as accurate observers. They proclaim, too, their statistics too much in the advertising style of quackery. This at least brings suspicion upon them; and then, sometimes, even the published statements of Homœopathic physicians in regard to their success, *have been proved to be false.* And besides, Homœopathists give us no definite statement of the principles on which their statistics in the cholera are collected.

This last point is one of great importance. When the cholera prevails, there are great numbers of cases of diarrhœa having such a proclivity to cholera, that we term the complaint *cholerinc.* Some of these cases end in real cholera. Others result in rather doubtful half-formed cases of the disease. But the great majority of them never are anything but cases of diarrhœa. Now the physician, who sets down in his statistics only undoubted cases, will make out different statistics altogether from those of the physician who includes the half-formed cases, and very widely different from those of the physician who reckons all cases of mere cholerine as true cases of cholera, and who thus makes out a large story of his success to appeal to the public credulity.

Homœopathists are not the only physicians who have made out large statistics of the cholera. The Eclectic physicians, as they style themselves, made some reports at a meeting of their National Association in Cincinnati, which even go beyond the statistics of Homœopathy. One physician, for example, reports five deaths in one hundred and fifty cases of cholera; another only three deaths in one hundred and fifty cases—another, but four deaths in seven hundred cases of all diseases—another, but two deaths in five hundred cases of all diseases, etc. I leave it to the Eclectics and the Homœopaths to settle their differences between themselves. Neither party, probably, believe the statistics of the other, while the community at large very generally disbelieve the statistics of both.

The same remarks substantially could be made in regard to all the other statistics of Homœopathy. They could be shown to be quite as unworthy of confidence as those which relate to the cholera. But it is not necessary. The cholera statistics, of which so much boast has been made, illustrate sufficiently the glaring defects, which mark all the statistics that are relied upon to prove the success of Homœopathic practice.

In this connection, I remark, that some of the popular ideas in regard to observation are very erroneous. Observation is considered a very easy work. It is only to see and hear, and that, it is supposed, can be done correctly by any one. But reasoning, on the other hand, is deemed to be difficult, and to require talent and skill to do it well. To say nothing here of the impropriety of this distinction so commonly made between observation and reasoning, it may be remarked, that in scientific investigation, the power of reasoning well is absolutely essential to good observation. If reason does not guide the observer, not only will his observations be confused and irrelevant, but the merest fancies will be mingled with them. The saying of Solomon, that "The wise man's eyes are in his head," is as true in science as it is in morals.

There has been quite as much poor observation in the world as poor reasoning. Good observers are of great value in science. They make all the discoveries. They relieve science of the rubbish with which theorizing observers, so often and so falsely called great reasoners, have encumbered it. In therapeutics, where there is so much liability to error, the difference between poor and good observation is more manifest than in relation to any other subject in the wide range of science. It is particularly true in medicine, both of professional and non-professional observation, that there is a great difference in the value of testimony coming from different witnesses, even when they testify simply in regard to what they have seen. It is said by some satirist—

> Optics sharp, it needs I ween,
> To see what is not to be seen.

Yet this has often been done in medicine by many Allopathists ; but more, abundantly more, by Homœopathists.

Let me illustrate in a very familiar manner the errors of observation to which I refer.

The descriptions given by non-professional ohservers of their personal experience, of what they have themselves felt, and seen, and heard, are often not only absurd, but laughable. A woman who had suffered from an inflammation in the foot, in describing her case, told me that she saw the inflammation move slowly down to the great toe, and then when it left the toe, it popped like a pistol. The reader of course does not believe the woman's statement. But why not ? She testified to what, as she believed, she actually saw and heard, and she was honest, and had eyes and ears capable in themselves of seeing and hearing correctly. You say that what she stated is impossible, and that she must have imagined it all. True ; and so do other observers, both common and professional, imagine that they see and hear, and their imaginings are often recorded as accurate observations. As the experience of the good woman corresponded with her notions, that is her theories, of disease, so is it with the false observations of more scientific theorizers. And though her experience was not only an impossibility, but a laughable one, it is on the face of it no more so than the experience of Hahnemann, when he describes a grotesque multitude of symptoms as produced by a decillionth of a grain of oystershell or common salt, or even by a single sniff from a phial containing a solitary infinitesimal globule. When he seriously notes down as the effects of some medicine such things as these—an itching, tickling sensation at the *outer* edge of the *palm* of the *left* hand, creeping in the upper lip and in the *point* of the nose, twitching in the cartilage of the ear, he winks, etc.—he forfeits his claim to our confidence in him as an observer, as really as the woman did, when she said that she saw the inflammation move down, and that when it went off she heard it pop like a pistol. The whole fifteen octavo volumes of Homœopathic provings are no more reliable than her statement, absurd as it is; and we are fully warranted in saying, that those who made these provings, and those who believe in them, and use them as guides in their practice, transgressing, as they do, the plainest rules of evidence, are not to be implicitly relied upon, even when they make statements in regard to what they have seen and heard.

Homœopathists complain that physicians are unwilling to apply to the claims of Homœopathy the test of their own experience. Professor Henderson says, that if they could be brought to do this, it would ensure its "universal adoption," because "for a rational man to try Homœopathy is tantamount to his conversion." But is this personal experience necessary? Must we go through with the provings upon ourselves, and observe the symptoms of the sick under the use of the globules, before we can decide whether Homœopathy be true? How is it with other doctrines? Do we feel obliged to test them all by our own experience? Can we not sometimes—do we not, and very properly, judge of the truth or falsity of a doctrine by other circumstances—the general character of those who believe it, the relations which it bears to known and long-established truths, and the character of the observations and reasonings by which it is attempted to be sustained? In this way we often see enough at the very threshold of an investigation to satisfy us without going any farther. Especially is this true when many minds have been engaged in developing and defending the doctrine, and in collecting and arranging the alleged facts upon which it is based. If in such a case, we find at the outset nothing but a mixture of inconsistent statements and loose analogies, we justly view it as a waste of time to put the new doctrine to the test of our own experience. Whether this conclusion be a correct one in regard to the doctrine called Homœopathy, the reader can judge from the exposition and examination of it which I have made in this essay.

But although the bare exposition of Homœopathy,

as it is presented to us by its advocates, is amply sufficient to show that it is false, and therefore the test of personal experience is wholly unnecessary, yet this test has been applied by Allopathists again and again. This has been done, both in regard to its provings and its treatment of the sick, by physicians of no doubtful character, as to their veracity and their competency as observers.

It is not my intention to introduce here all the evidence which I have been able to collect. A few examples only will be sufficient.

Many physicians have "proved" Cinchona or Peruvian bark; and though this, as the reader will remember, is the article whose effects are said to have given to Hahnemann the first idea of the great central doctrine of his system, they have not found that it has produced the symptoms ascribed to it by him. It seems to have no "affinity" for those who are not diseased with the Hahnemannic mania. M. Double, a physician of the highest character in Paris, as long ago as 1801, before he had heard of Homœopathy, experimented with some friends to ascertain the effects of Cinchona. They took it in all kinds of doses for four months, but none of them had any "totality" of symptoms similar to that which is presented in intermittent fever. And M. Bonnet, President of the Royal Society of Medicine, of Bourdeaux, observed that soldiers who took Cinchona as a preventive of disease, never experienced those effects, which Homœopathists, committed to a "foregone conclusion," so uniformly experience on taking it in their "provings." M. Andral, one of the best practical observers in medicine that France has produced, experimented in connection with several persons in health with Cinchona, Aconite, etc., during the space of a whole year, and the provings of Homœopathists were not verified by these trials in the slightest degree. In 1835, the following proposition was made to the most prominent Homœopathist in Paris, viz.—that he should select ten remedies and prepare them himself, and that one of these, chosen by lot, should be administered to him, and then that he should afterward, at such time as pleased him, come forward and state which of the ten substances he had taken. He was not willing to try the experiment. And yet no one can say that this would not be a perfectly fair mode of testing the provings.

Of the trials of Homœopathic remedies upon the sick, I shall only notice that very thorough and long-continued one which was made by Andral. This "eminent and very enlightened Allopathist," as the Homœopathic Examiner once called him, made this statement in 1835, to the Academy of Medicine. "I have submitted this doctrine to experiment; I can reckon at this time from one hundred and thirty to one hundred and forty cases recorded with perfect fairness in a great hospital, under the eye of numerous witnesses; to avoid every objection, I obtained my remedies of M. Guibourt, who keeps a Homœopathic pharmacy, and whose strict exactness is well known;

the regimen has been scrupulously observed, and I obtained from the sisters attached to the hospital, a special regimen, such as Hahnemann orders. I was told, however, some months since, that I had not been faithful to all the rules of the doctrine. I therefore took the trouble to begin again; I have studied the practice of the Parisian Homœopathists, as I had studied their books, and I became convinced that they treated their patients as I had treated mine; and I affirm that I have been as rigorously exact as any other person." Though these trials were made with such boasted articles as Cinchona, Aconite, Belladonna, etc., yet Andral says that he could not see that they produced any effect. He administered Aconite in more than forty cases marked by those feverish symptoms which, according to Homœopathists, it so uniformly removes; but he could not perceive the slightest effect upon the pulse or upon the temperature of the skin in any of these cases.

"These statements look pretty honest," as Dr. Holmes says; and, coming from a man so eminently "rational" as Andral is, they show that Professor Henderson, was somewhat in error in saying, that "for a rational man to try Homœopathy is tantamount to his conversion."

CHAPTER VI.

ESTIMATE OF HAHNEMANN.

Having examined the system of doctrine and practice put forth by Hahnemann, it will be interesting to look at the character of its author.

Hahnemann cannot be said to be an impostor in the strictest sense of that word. He was for the most part undoubtedly sincere in his belief.* He may have had occasionally some faltering of his faith; but generally it was firm and enthusiastic. He became an errorist just as multitudes before him had done. He narrowed his views down to a certain set of facts, of which he fancied that he had discovered the explanation. And the more he thought, the more did the subject grow in his mind. The result was, that this explanation, this theory, became to him the sun of his

* In saying that Hahnemann was for the most part sincere in the belief of his doctrines, I must not be understood to mean that he was an honest man. His selling common borax as a newly discovered salt for a *louis d'or* per ounce, of which sin there is no evidence that ever he repented, shows that morally he was a *cheat*. But this is not at all inconsistent with his cheating himself into a sincere belief of the delusions which his busy fancy had conjured up in his mind.

system. It was the only true light, and it made everything clear to his vision. The spirit of delusion was now fully upon him, and it blinded him to all facts which were plainly inconsistent with his all-absorbing idea. The thought too, that he had made a great discovery, intoxicated him. He was a medical fanatic. He was the victim of what might be termed a scientific insanity; and he went on from one delusion to another, till at length no absurdity was too monstrous for his belief. His psoric theory, the climax of all medical absurdities, shows a height of delusion which has seldom been reached by the human mind.

It is interesting and instructive to watch the movements of a mind of which the spirit of delusion has taken possession. It is not a mind, you will observe, that is simply in error from partial views and hasty inferences. This latter is a state from which the mind can recover. But not so with the condition of mind to which I refer. In this case there is a radical defect—a mental disease, from which there can be no recovery except by a thorough change of the mental habits. Not even the casting out of cherished errors will do it. This would be only cutting off the branches, while the root and body of the evil remained to put forth other, and perhaps stronger, branches in their place. The admission of one fallacy, if the mind become enamored with it, prepares for the admission of other fallacies. And as the power of estimating the value of evidence becomes more and more impaired, each fallacy is commonly more gross than the one which preceded it. Thus it was with the mind of Hahnemann. Once in the power of the spirit of delusion, it became after a little time ready for the reception of all kinds of error. To his own medical errors Hahnemann added a belief to the full in mesmerism* and clairvoyance, with all their mummeries and juggleries ; and if he were living at this day, such impostures as Davis' revelations would have received his implicit confidence, and even that grossest of all delusions, the pretended communication with the spiritual world by "*rappings*," would have been believed as readily as the efficacy of infinitesimal globules.

One of the peculiarities in the workings of Hahnemann's mind is very remarkable. I refer to his coming to the most stupendous conclusions without seeming to note or even to know when and how he did it. Most discoverers of great truths tell us, and very minutely, by what processes of observation and reasoning they made their discoveries. But Hahnemann announces what he claims to be discoveries, and those too of the most astounding character ; and yet he informs us of the manner in which his mind was led on to its conclusions, only in relation to a single one of them, viz.—the doctrine, *similia similibus curantur*. The doctrine of the efficacy of infinitesimal doses, which, if it be true, is one of the most wonderful truths which was ever discovered, was first announced, as I have already stated, in a note, and

See Organon, p. 294 and 203, and Materia Medica Pura, vol i. p. 21.

that only incidentally ; and we are no where informed at what time and under what circumstances the 'discovery' was made. One would suppose that a discovery which makes a grain of any medicine sufficient to supply all the inhabitants of the earth centuries, nay, ages upon ages, with all the doses which they would need of that article, would have a date in the mind of its discoverer, and would be reckoned as an era in medicine ; and that the circumstances which led to its discovery would be minutely detailed in every notice of it. But no. So stilly did the mountain-mind of Hahnemann bring forth this "ridiculus mus," as it has shown itself to be, that no record seems to have been made of the period of its birth.

All theorizers have been disposed to fix upon some one doctrine or principle as the centre of a system. To the speculative mind there is a fascination in the idea of discovering a single key to the explanation of a wide range of phenomena. Hence we have the *archeus* of Van Helmont, the *anima* of Stahl, the *excitability* of Brown, the *gastro-enterite* of Broussais, the *unity of disease* of Rush, and a multitude of favorite doctrines that have had their day in the medical world. So too, Samuel Thompson was governed by the same disposition, when he adopted as the centre of his system the doctrine, that heat is life, and Samuel Hahnemann, when he fancied that in *similia similibus curantur* he had found the magic key which would unlock all the secrets of therapeutics.

The folly of Homœopathy is preëminently a "folly in wisdom hatch'd." Hahnemann was in some senses a wise man, though not in the best sense in which that word is used. He had some talent, though by no means of a high order. His ingenuity was fruitful; but it was so blind, that he could never avoid exposing the weak points of his argument, and he was constantly stumbling, without knowing it, over the grossest inconsistencies. He had no true scientific acumen. He analyzed nothing with any discrimination. He was incapable of detecting a fallacy, and the loosest analogies were to him sound arguments.

Professor Henderson in apologizing for his errors, which he seems to think are quite trivial, speaks of him as belonging to a class of men who have an "ardent genius," and who "do not always wait for the tardy steps of induction; but as the history of almost all the great discoveries, as well as of the great errors of genius, declares, grasp by anticipation at conclusions which future experience is left to confirm or annul." But Henderson in his blind admiration entirely mistakes the character of Hahnemann's mind. It had none of the attributes of the discoverer. Free to suppose, it could never prove. It could dream, and it believed its dreams to be realities. If it anticipated in its dreams what experience would afterward "confirm," it would be only by stumbling upon it by mere chance.

No discoverer ever had such a mind as Hahnemann's. Newton, with whom Hahnemann is often compared by his admirers, had a mind of an entirely different cast. Hahnemann dreamed, but Newton thought. Both supposed ; but Hahnemann called his suppositions facts, while Newton "waited for the tardy steps of induction" to test his suppositions. "I shall not mingle conjectures with certainties," said Newton ; but Hahnemann did nothing but conjecture, and deemed all his conjectures to be certainties. "The tardy steps of induction," Hahnemann never trod. Yet they are steps which are absolutely necessary to the establishment of any important truth. If Hahnemann has really discovered any such truths, he has done it by a process different from that of all other discoverers.

Place Hahnemann then, if you will, among the theorizers of "ardent genius" that have from time to time made the world to wonder; but insult not science by ranking him among the noble discoverers of her hidden treasures. He only had visions of imaginary treasures, and lived in his visions as if they were realities. He was but a wild dreamer in science. And when he began to dream there was no limit to the illusions with which he was enchanted. Farther and farther did he depart from the truth. More and more erratic and absurd were his vagaries. A long life did he live, and he filled up the measure of his folly by that most absurd of all human conceptions, the psoric theory.

Talent and learning may serve either wisdom or folly. When they serve wisdom, it is a "reasonable service;" but when folly, they perform a slavish service, and that abundantly and unremittingly. And though folly never appears so ridiculous as when thus attended, never is it so insensible to its real position—never is it so blind to the truth, and so obstinate in pursuing its purpose. The folly of an ignorant man may be removed by enlightening his ignorance; but a "wit turned fool" is seldom converted from his folly. Once set out in his career of delusion, though he be the laughing-stock of all sensible people, as he so proudly displays the ingeniously-wrought, but flimsy gewgaws with which he is be-decked, he is never awakened to a conviction of his folly, but keeps on in his career to the end. Thus was it with Hahnemann, who may justly be termed the prince of scientific fools, as Paracelsus was the prince of quacks.

The character of Hahnemann is impressed to a great extent upon his followers. Minds of a particular cast have been attracted by the Homœopathic delusion, and they have imbibed most fully the spirit of their great exemplar. They are not minds which have "the calm and cautious spirit of philosophy" so falsely claimed for Hahnemann by Mr. Marmaduke Sampson. The advocates of Homœopathy, like its author, are dreamers, and not thinkers. Among them all there is not to be found one that can be called an accurate, reliable observer, and a sound reasoner. The literature of Homœopathy, therefore, is made up of flimsy reasonings and loose analogies. Most of it has not even the merit of ingenuity. Even those works which are at all ingenious, present us with an abundance of glaring inconsistencies and ridiculous trivialities. Sampson exhibits more talent than any other author on Homœopathy that I have consulted; and yet his book so far from being marked with "the calm and cautious spirit of philosophy," is a tissue of misrepresentations and fallacies. Joslin's book certainly shows some smartness; but every page contains evidences of his utter want of a discriminating judgment, and of plain common sense. And as to the common herd of Homœopathic writers, the talent which they exhibit, like their doses, is very dilute and infinitesimal in amount. The whole field of Homœopathic literature is a barren waste, covered with a dry and stinted vegetation, with here and there a flaunting but fruitless flower.*

The manner in which Homœopathy has been treated by the medical profession, has been the subject of severe comment on the part of Hahnemann's followers. That its reception has not been at all flattering, is universally acknowledged. It has been adopted by an exceedingly small fraction of the pro-

* Most of the controversial literature of Homœopathy is really contemptible. I refer the reader to Dr. Wosselhoeft's letters in reply to Dr. Holmes' capital lectures on Homœopathy and its kindred delusions, as an example. This pamphlet of fifty pages is vapid and irrelevant throughout, and not a page of it merits the name of a reply. It certainly must tax the patience of "the benevolent reader," to whom he dedicates it, to read it through. If I understand the application of the motto on his title page—*Many are called but few are chosen*; it is ridiculously impudent as well as shockingly profane.

fession—so small, that as a body they may be fairly said to reject it. And of this fraction only a very few are above mediocrity in point of talent, and these have that peculiar cast of mind which renders them prone to delusion. In our own country it is very well known that no physician of any commanding influence has been converted to Homœopathy, although Sampson says that, "the theatre of its widest reception is found to be amongst the shrewdest, the most practical, and, on other than national points, the least prejudiced people upon earth—the inhabitants of the United States."* And in Great Britain, I believe the

* It is a little amusing to see how American Homœopathists boast of the success of their system in Europe; and then again, how European Homœopathists proclaim, on their side of the water, its triumphs in this country. These references to places at a distance are quite convenient sometimes. False statements about matters at home are too easily corrected to be made available. Homœopathists seem to be aware of this. Their large stories about the rapid advances of Hahnemannism, generally refer to distant places or other countries. It takes some time and costs some trouble therefore, to prove their falsity. But it has been done in many cases, and I will give a single example. The following announcement was made in a French journal—"By a decree of October, 1841, the Emperor of Austria has created a chair of Homœopathy in the faculty of Vienna; named M.M. Worm and Nerbar, professors, and appropriated one hundred beds in the St. Elizabeth Hospital for the Homœopathic treatment of diseases, under the superintendence of Dr. Levy." One would hardly think that so circumstantial a statement would be made if it were not true. But it turns out to be untrue in every particular. Dr. Sigmund, a distinguished physician of Vienna, who was sent by his government to France to study the organization of the medical profession in that country, on seeing the above statement, published a contradiction of it, in which he says—"It has never been proposed to create a *chair* of Homœopathy in the

only Allopathic physician of any pretensions to eminence, that has become a Homœopathist, is Dr. Henderson, and he has so great a mental obliquity, that he apologizes laboriously for Hahnemann's psoric theory, and shows that he well nigh believes it.

And in Germany also, the land of its birth, Homœopathy has made but few converts from the ranks of the profession. In 1835, when it was much more flourishing in that country than it now is, at a meeting of physicians numbering over six hundred, Homœopathy, on being introduced to their notice by some member, was at once scouted as unworthy of a moment's attention.

Homœopathy has been fairly before medical men for fifty years; and the profession has passed its verdict upon it in the most deliberate and positive manner. Some are disposed to think that this verdict is good for nothing, and openly charge medical men, as a body, with a wilful blindness to the truth of Homœopathy. If this charge be well founded, the medical profession are governed in relation to this doctrine by a spirit altogether different from that which they have manifested towards all other new doctrines and opinions. Look over the whole history of medi-

faculty of Vienna; neither have the government enacted an order to create a *clinique* of this kind. The hospital mentioned is one closed to students and strangers; a distinct foundation, served by the sisters of St. Elizabeth. and the physician of which is one of our brethren, Dr. Weninger, who has never practiced Homœopathy. M.M. Worm, Nerbar, and Levy, are entirely unknown in Vienna."

cine, and observe the course which the profession have pursued in regard to the numberless doctrines and theories which have arisen from time to time. As they have passed away one after another, they have been examined and sifted by medical men, and while much has been rejected, much has been retained and added to the permanent treasures of our science. And you cannot adduce a single instance, in which anything that time has shown to be valuable, has not in a very short period gained a strong hold upon the professional mind, however great might be the opposition to it at its first promulgation. If Homœopathy be truly valuable, it is the first thing of this character which has failed to be thus established among medical men. It is a single solitary exception, showing an irrational obstinacy which the profession have certainly not been wont to manifest.*

The first reception of a doctrine does not at all indicate its value. Some groundless doctrines have had a wide popularity at the outset in the profession; while others which are founded in truth have been comparatively slow in becoming established. The true and rational judgment of the profession in regard to any doctrine cannot be obtained at once. Minds in every quarter and of every cast must scrutinize the evidences on which it is based. We must wait a lit-

* The assertion so often and so boldly made by Homœopathists, that the profession rejected the discoveries of Harvey and Jenner, just as they now reject Homœopathy, is utterly false. See "Medical Delusions," p. 77.

tle, and at length a reliable verdict is rendered. If there be any truth in the doctrine, whatever there is, is found, and is preserved, while what is untrue is rejected. If the doctrine, on the other hand, be entirely untrue, though it may prevail for a time, it soon passes away. And if any doctrine meet from the first with a steady rejection on the part of the great body of the profession, notwithstanding its claims have been perseveringly urged by its advocates, this is very good evidence against its truth.

This verdict, then, of a multiform and accumulated experience is an indication of value, which is by no means to be disregarded. And the farther science is advanced, the greater is the reliance which can be placed upon this verdict or settled opinion of scientific bodies of men. It should of course be much more readily relied upon now than when science was encumbered with errors, and was retarded in its progress by an undue reverence for antiquity. Even then this sifting process of an extended and varied experience was applied to every new doctrine, but not with so much faithfulness and discrimination as it is at the present day.

Let me be fairly understood. I am no advocate for a blind and implicit obedience to authorities in science. But the opinions of men who are competent to judge, when they have had sufficient time and opportunity for judging, are surely of some value as evidence. Especially is this true when great numbers of such men, constituting scientific bodies, have given their opinions, both individually and collectively, and have adhered to them for a great length of time. This has been done in relation to Homœopathy for the last fifty years. All the evidence which has been presented in regard to this doctrine during all this time has fastened the conviction upon the profession, that it is false and absurd. And let it be remembered, that the profession which thus so perseveringly and almost universally reject Homœopathy is composed of men who have every variety of opinions, and are not bound together by any particular set of doctrines. There is another circumstance also that gives significance to this rejection of Homœopathy. I refer to the fact that, while so few physicians have become Homœopathists, the great majority of those who practise according to this system are poorly educated and irresponsible men. Unable to get any hold upon the profession, Homœopathy has received most of its votaries from the people; and being rejected by the schools of medicine, it has made a show of getting up schools of its own.

Let us suppose, now, a parallel case. Suppose that fifty years ago some theologian had broached a new mode of biblical interpretation, which, if true, would set aside all old rules and modes, as Hahnemann's system, if true, would do in medicine—that, though the author of this system was a talented man, few among all the regularly educated divines had adopted it—that of this number but a very few were men of any standing—that the great majority of those who proclaimed the new doctrine were poorly-educated men, and that this new sect opposed themselves to all "regular" theologians of every name, and set up schools to supply the community with divines, who are educated in nothing but the absurdities of their system. Would it not, I ask, be claimed of us laymen, that we should believe, almost as a matter of course from the very reception thus given to the new doctrine by theologians, that it was false? Would it not be said, that it is not to be supposed that theologians, with all their various differences, would unite as a body in rejecting what is truly valuable; and that if the doctrine had any truth in it, it could certainly get a lodgment in some of all the various theological schools, and that schools need not therefore be instituted purposely for its propagation?

The parallel is complete in this case. It is not defective in a single particular; and yet if we should assert that the rejection of this new mode of interpretation for fifty years by theologians as a body is no evidence against its truth, it would be taking the same ground that many clergymen take in relation to the rejection on the part of physicians of Hahnemann's mode of interpreting disease and its cure.

Let us take a parallel case of a different character. Suppose that some political fanatic comes forward with an entirely new interpretation of the constitution, which, as it conflicts with all established principles of interpretation, is rejected by jurists and statesmen as a body throughout the country, and that only here and there one can be found that adopts it. And suppose that this rejection of the new doctrine continues, and that in the lapse of fifty years it does not gain a foothold, among educated lawyers and statesmen, though it may have a multitude of uneducated advocates. Such a state of things, all will allow, furnishes good evidence against the truth of the doctrine, for the plain reason, that the opinion of those who are most competent to judge on the subject is worthy of respect and confidence.

The same parallel can be drawn in regard to any science or any subject. Public opinion in scientific bodies of men, when ample time has been given for its due establishment, has always commanded respect; and why, I ask, should an exception be made in regard to medicine? Is the medical profession less entitled to confidence than other scientific bodies? Are its deliberate verdicts to be contemned as worthless? This is claimed not only by ignorant radicals, but even by some men who are esteemed by the community as being preëminent in wisdom and goodness. They maintain that physicians *will not* see the evidences of the success of Homœopathy, and that they reject it from motives of interest, mingled with an overweaning attachment to old and established opinions. We think that they can hardly be aware of the foulness of the aspersion which they thus cast upon our profession. If what they say is true, physicians are an exceedingly inhumane class of men—they are continually sacrificing the health and even the lives of their patients to a wicked prejudice.*

* The fact that many clergymen of eminence have taken this ground,

Homœopathy appears before us in a somewhat singular position. It pushes its claims in a manner different from that of any other system or theory, which, like this, has originated in the profession. The advocates of all other systems have endeavored to propagate their doctrines among medical men alone. They did not even establish schools for the special purpose of disseminating their opinions, but sought to introduce them into the schools already in existence. Neither Brown nor Broussais, for example, founded schools to teach their doctrines, although they were so different from the opinions which prevailed in the profession. All founders of systems previous to Hahnemann endeavored to leaven the whole profession, caring little comparatively for the opinions of the unprofessional public. But the advocates of Homœopathy, instead of seeking to change the opinions of medical men alone, appeal to the public against the profession, and aim at establishing another medical profession in opposition to that already in existence. And for this purpose they have instituted schools in order to indoctrinate the disciples of the new system in its principles.

has materially lessened the confidence which medical men generally have in their learning and judgment. When, in addition to giving credence to such an absurdity as Homœopathy, against the plainest rules of evidence, they cast such a false imputation upon our profession, it is not strange that physicians are ready to infer, that they are as irrational and as regardless of the true rules of evidence on theological as they are on medical subjects. Scepticism has often thus been encouraged, not to say engendered, and a respect for our holy religion has been destroyed by this conduct on the part of its ministers.

Homœopathy, therefore, is mongrel in its character. While it has a scientific air, and puts forth the most ostentatious scientific pretensions, it comes before us very much in the guise of quackery, and it uses all the appliances of quackery to gain the popular favor.* And more than this, while it imprudently claims to be the only true system of medicine, it leaves all researches in physiology, and in anatomy, both natural and morbid, to those whom it denounces, as obstinately clinging to antiquated errors.

Homœopathy and its sister delusion, Thompsonianism, strongly resemble each other in the manner in which they prosecute their claims. Though they move in different spheres, their tactics are very much the same. Though

*Dr. Blatchford, in his witty and excellent address on Homœopathy, thus remarks: Another peculiar feature in Homœopathy, not much calculated to give it success with the thinking community, is that their periodicals and other organs, animate and inanimate, speak of no *unsuccessful application* of their principles: none but palpable cases of cure are mentioned, and these are served up in a dress to suit the multitude. This is a feature which is certainly calculated to ally Homœopathy with empiricism, to say the least; and reminds one of the artful contrivance of the proprietor of a certain mineral spring in England, who kept one room in which were deposited the crutches of all those patients who had received so much benefit from the waters as not to require their assistance any longer. One day a company of ladies and gentlemen, as usual, were shown into this apartment, with its hundreds of crutches, and the virtues of the waters highly extolled, when an old decrepid servant of the establishment, who was seated in one corner of the room, said in a low tone to a gentleman who stood near, "Ah me! they take good care to say nothing about the heaps of crutches we burn up every year of the poor creatures who come here only to die. Dead bones tell no tales, you know."

Homœopathy may look with contempt upon the coarse radicalism of her vulgar and ignorant sister, she has the same radicalism in a more refined and specious form. Both cry out against the "regular" profession; and the tendency of the efforts of both, however stoutly the genteel and learned patrons of Homœopathy may deny it, is to destroy the safeguards which secure to the community a well-educated body of medical men. Other systems, as Chrono-Thermalism, Eclecticism, etc., have also arisen, and have taken the fashion of their measures from Hahnemannism and Thompsonism, and have joined with them in the great work of medical radicalism.

CHAPTER VII.

CONCLUDING OBSERVATIONS.

I WILL conclude this essay with a few remarks upon some of the lessons which both the medical profession and the community may draw from this exposure of Homœopathy.

The profession may learn from the fantasies of Hahnemannn the evils which result to science from a disposition to theorize. There is no one thing that has so much retarded the progress of medicine as this disposition, which has been so prevalent among medical men in all ages and countries. Ingenious hypotheses have, to a very great extent, taken the place of accurate and extended observations in the past records of our science. And as we look back upon the history of medicine, and scan the influence of all the prominent men in our profession in all past times, we can see in the case of each that his usefulness was in an inverse ratio to his disposition to theorize. It is the men of observation, who have been content to tread "the tardy steps of induction," instead of taking the airy flights of theory, that have gathered the real treasures of medical science. Theorists have never done this, except when they have ceased to theorize, and begun to observe. Now, Hahnemann never did any thing but theorize. He was under the entire dominion of the theorizing spirit. His was no partial possession. And it must be remembered that the difference between him and other theorists is one chiefly of degree. They have not, I allow, wandered as far away from the truth as he did; but so far as they have gone, it was upon the same track of delusion. This being the case, the example of Hahnemann can well be cited, as showing the legitimate tendencies of the theorizing spirit, when unrestrained and carried out to their full extent.

The investigation of Homœopathy which we have gone through in this essay, is of advantage, not merely in exposing the falsity of this vaunted system, but in developing and illustrating the rules or principles of evidence, which should be applied in testing the value of any remedy or any system of practice. The errors which have been committed by the believers in Homœopathy, in the application of these principles, are not new and singular; but they arise from the same sources with the multitude of errors that have prevailed in relation to all other systems and remedies. The exposition, therefore, which I have made of the absurdities and inconsistencies of Homœopathy, may, by revealing the common sources of medical errors generally, be of some service in correcting that loose habit of mind which is so prevalent both in the profession and in the community, in regard to evidence on the subject of medicine.

On this point there is great need of a reform, even among medical men. The same principles of evidence which reject Homœopathic observation as inconclusive and false, must, if rigidly applied, reject a large portion of the observations contained in the annals of medicine. Too much has been taken upon trust, without regard to the degree of fidelity or capacity in the observer. A sifting process needs to be applied to the recorded experience of the profession. The principles upon which causes are indisputably connected with their results need to be thoroughly examined, and the difficulties in their application to be faithfully developed, that they may be justly appreciated. And the gross errors of Homœopathists in this respect, may serve to direct the attention of medical men to their own lesser errors, and to the cautions which are requisite in estimating the effects of remedies.

Medicine has nothing to fear from pushing the rules of evidence to their strictest application, though very much of the recorded experience of physicians may be demolished, or be brought under suspicion. Even if we discard all that is in the least doubtful, there is enough left to establish medicine as a science, and that, too, a science not barren and meagre, but abounding in facts and principles.

Another lesson, which may be learned from Homœopathy by the profession, is the importance of observing the operations of nature in her efforts to remove disease. The cures which are effected under *true* Homœopathic treatment, are not effected by medicine, but by nature, sometimes with the aid of mental influence. The experience, therefore, which is presented by Homœopathy, of which physicians occasionally obtain some glimpses, is of much value, as showing the power of nature to cure disease, and developing the principles upon which she acts in doing it. It is in this way that the most absurd of all medical delusions may be made to do essential service to the cause of science and humanity.

It has sometimes been claimed by the advocates of Homœopathy, that Hahnemann has been the great teacher to our profession of the lesson to which I have referred. It is not only a false but an impudent claim. Not only did he never teach it directly, but he proclaimed a doctrine, as the reader has seen in a former part of this essay, in direct opposition to it, and in every way cast contempt upon the curative powers of nature in comparison with the effects of his infinitesimal globules. And more than this; the lesson had begun to be learned by medical men from other sources, before Homœopathy was known. It was learned from the *expectant* mode of treatment, which has been so long popular with the French. It was learned in the individual experience of multitudes of physicians, who found Sydenham's experience in the treatment of the small-pox to be verified to a great extent in other diseases. And for more than half a century, there has been a decided movement in the profession in opposition to an indiscriminate heroic medication. This movement has been becoming every year more and more general. And the utmost that can be said of Homœopathy on this point is, that it has had a decided influence, though an indirect one, in favoring this tendency in the profession.

Dr. Forbes, in remarking upon the present prevalence of indiscriminate and profuse medication in the profession, not only overstates the truth, but is inconsistent with himself in other parts of his essay, in which he speaks of the advance which has been made in practical medicine. His language is : "Things have arrived at such a pitch, that they cannot be worse. They must mend or end." Even upon his own showing, things have been worse. They have been most obviously mending, and that for a long time. If we compare the therapeutics of the present day with that which prevailed fifty or an hundred years ago, medication is vastly more cautious and discriminating than it was then, and the movements of nature, in the cure of disease, are much more narrowly observed. And, at this time, there are multitudes of minds in the profession on the right track in their inquiries ; and we have reason to anticipate that great advances will now be rapidly made in the practical part of our science.

While the change which I have indicated is going on in the profession, it is an interesting and important inquiry for each individual practitioner, what course he ought to pursue in his own private practice? Must he wait and do almost nothing till he can find out all the truth? Because "*heroic*" medicines have done so much harm, must he for the present utterly forbear using them? This would be going to the opposite extreme, and, in his endeavor to be certain of doing no harm, he would surely sometimes lose rich opportunities of doing good. The experience of every judicious physician, even if all cases in the least degree doubtful be left out of view, testifies most clearly to the fact, that there are times when powerful remedies can do much good. And the more discriminating he is, the more skillful of course will he be in discovering the times and the circumstances which call for their application. The duty of the practitioner plainly is to use in each case all the means which his judgment dictates; at the same time he should learn all that he can, by watching narrowly the effects of his remedies, and by comparing his own experience with that of other reliable observers. If physicians as a body would engage in this rigid observation of the influence of remedies upon disease, while a large portion of the positive medication still remaining would be discarded, great triumphs would be achieved in the discriminate use of heroic remedies, which now we fail to achieve, because with our present dim and confused experience, we so often fail to perceive the modes, and mark the times, in which they should be applied.

That there is still prevalent in the profession a lamentable carelessness in the observation of the effects of remedies is evident, from the readiness with which every new remedy or mode of practice obtains a currency among medical men, before there is really time to test its merits. This mushroom popularity could not attend every new thing which is introduced to the notice of medical men, if rigid and patient observation were a general habit in the profession, instead of being confined, as it now is, to a comparatively small portion of its members.

The enemies of our profession have been exceedingly busy in pointing out its defects and errors. And none have been more active in this work than Homœopathists. They seem to prize such exposures as the very best arguments which can be adduced in favor of their own system; as if, forsooth, because Allopathy has defects and inconsistencies, therefore Homœopathy must be true. However provoking this may be, it is the part of wisdom to take good-naturedly all such attacks, and profit, so far as we can by any discoveries which our enemies may make of our deficiencies.

In noticing a few of the lessons which the community may learn from this exposure of Homœopathy I must be brief.

Homœopathy adds another to the multitude of illustrations of the facility with which the community may be deceived in relation to the comparative results of different remedies and modes of practice. There is no remedy, and no mode of practice, that has not obtained for a time a high reputation for success. And this has been true of those which after-experience has shown to be valueless, as well as those that have had some ground for their reputation. This being the case, it might reasonably be expected, that the community would learn wisdom from this experience, which has been so often repeated, and that the history of past delusions would serve to guard them against yielding a ready credence to those of the present day. But this is a lesson which they are slow to learn. And hence the necessity of that thorough and patient examination, which we have made in this essay, of one of the most absurd delusions that ever entered the human mind.

The evidences, upon which the pretensions of Homœopathy, as a system of practice, are based, are precisely of the same loose character with those upon which the alleged success of Perkins' Tractors, the royal touch, the tar-water of Bishop Berkeley, or any other of the multitude of past quackeries has been predicated.* It is time that intelligent men should understand the fallacy of these evidences. It is time that they should be aware of the special necessity there is for a rigid application of the rules of evidence in medical experience; and they should demand that every new doctrine or remedy should be subjected to

* For a full presentation of this subject, see "Medical Delusions.

the thorough test of a careful and extended observation, instead of receiving it, as they now often do, on proofs of the slightest and narrowest character.

The most important lesson which needs to be learned by the community is in relation to their duty of sustaining the medical profession. It is obviously as true of medicine, as it is of any other science, that its advancement can be best promoted by securing for the work of its investigation a well educated body of men. And any encouragement which is accorded to quackery in any form, or to any sect which comes out in opposition to the regular profession, tends to defeat this desirable object. It is a strange policy which would make an exception of medical science in this respect. Medical men do not differ so much from other bodies of scientific men, as to need the appliances of quackery in order to establish any thing that is valuable. They are not, as a body, bound down by a stupid and obstinate attachment to antiquated customs and notions. They are quite as ready as the votaries of other sciences to welcome every new discovery or invention. And further than this, though quackery has flourished in all ages, and has boasted itself mightily of its achievements, I know of not one of all the discoveries and improvements that have been made in medicine to which quackery has the shadow of a claim.

The true position of the advocates of Homœopathy should be understood. They attack both the science and the profession of medicine. Lofty and scientific as are their pretensions, their spirit is the very spirit of radicalism. They aim, as do the advocates of other exclusive and absurd systems, less refined and elaborate than this, to destroy the medical profession, and to substitute in its place a mere sect, bound together by an ephemeral folly, and founded by one who began his career as an open and unblushing quack.

In view of the above considerations, we ask the intelligent and influential in the community to decide whether they will consent to encourage this radicalism in medicine, or whether they will unite in throwing around our profession all those safe-guards which are needed to secure its advancement, and to enable it to deliver society from the evils of quackery. The issue is distinct and clear. Every man's influence is thrown into the one scale or the other. It is not a light thing that a man does, who gives his countenance to delusion and quackery, even though it be but a momentary act, and an exception to his ordinary treatment of the medical profession. He lends by this act his sanction to the whole system of imposture, which the opposers of a well-educated profession, from Hahnemann down to the most ignorant of village quacks, or the basest seller of patent nostrums, are endeavoring to foist upon the community.

It is no small consideration that the influence of this issue extends beyond our science and our profession. The radicalism, which is so thoughtlessly encouraged by so many of even the good and intelligent of the community to make its attacks upon us, is thus emboldened in its warfare against other interests, even against that most precious of all interests, the best gift of God to man, the religion of the Bible. Such tendencies as this, surely every good citizen, every lover of science, of good order, of morality, of religion, should resist in every form in which they may appear.

LIST OF HOMŒOPATHIC AUTHORITIES REFERRED TO IN THIS ESSAY.

Hahnemann's Organon, ...	. *Dublin*, 1833.
Hahnemann's Materia Medica Pura, . .	*New York*, 1846.
Stapf's Materia Medica, ...	*New York*, 1846.
Jahr's Manual. "Translated from the German, by authority of the North American Academy of the Homœopathic Healing Art," .	. . 1838.
Henderson's Inquiry, ...	*New York*, 1846
Homœopathy, its Principle, Theory, and Practice, by Marmaduke B. Sampson, . .	. *London*, 1848.
Hull's Laurie, ...	*New York*, 1848.
Hartmann's Homœopathic Remedies, . .	*Philadelphia*, 1841.
Marcy's Homœopathic Theory and Practice of Medicine, ...	*New York*, 1850.
Hering's Domestic Physician, . . .	*Philadelphia*, 1845.
Joslin's Principles of Homœopathy, . .	*New York*, 1850.

Besides these, there are various pamphlets issued from time to time, and some numbers of different Homœopathic periodicals.

www.ingramcontent.com/pod-product-compliance
Lightning Source LLC
LaVergne TN
LVHW021405110826
845150LV00007B/1799

* 9 7 8 1 4 2 5 5 1 2 1 6 3 *